Hepatitis B and C Management and Treatment

Thierry Poynard
Service d'Hépato-Gastroentérologie
Groupe Hospitalier Pitié-Salpêtrière
Paris
France

MARTIN DUNITZ

© 2002 Martin Dunitz Ltd, a member of the Taylor & Francis group

First published in the United Kingdom in 2002
by Martin Dunitz Ltd, The Livery House, 7–9 Pratt Street, London NW1 0AE

Tel.:   +44 (0) 20 7482 2202
Fax.:   +44 (0) 20 7267 0159
E-mail: info.dunitz@tandf.co.uk
Website: http://www.dunitz.co.uk

Although every effort has been made to ensure that drug doses and other information are presented accurately in this publication, the ultimate responsibility rests with the prescribing physician. Neither the publishers nor the authors can be held responsible for errors or for any consequences arising from the use of information contained herein. For detailed prescribing information or instructions on the use of any product or procedure discussed herein, please consult the prescribing information or instructional material issued by the manufacturer.

A CIP record for this book is available from the British Library.

ISBN 1-84184-077-7

Distributed in the USA by
Fulfilment Center
Taylor & Francis
7625 Empire Drive
Florence, KY 41042, USA
Toll Free Tel: 1-800-634-7064
E-mail: cserve@routledge_ny.com

Distributed in Canada by
Taylor & Francis
74 Rolark Drive
Scarborough
Ontario M1R 4G2, Canada
Toll Free Tel: 1-877-226-2237
E-mail: tal_fran@istar.ca

Distributed in the rest of the world by
ITPS Limited
Cheriton House
North Way, Andover
Hampshire SP10 5BE, UK
Tel: +44 (0) 1264 332424
E-mail: reception@itps.co.uk

Composition by Wearset Ltd, Boldon, Tyne and Wear
Printed and bound in Great Britain by Cromwell Press Ltd.

Contents

About the author

Thierry Poynard completed his medical training at the University of Paris South in 1976. He received his PhD in Biostatistics in 1986 and completed his internship and residency training at the Hôpitaux Assistance Publique, Paris, in 1980. He was visiting Assistant Professor at the UCLA Medical Center in 1983, and has been Professor of Gastroenterology at the Groupe Hospitalier Pitié-Salpêtrière since 1993.

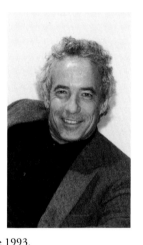

Professor Poynard is the author of over 240 original publications, including a number on ground-breaking investigations. These include the use of propranolol for the prevention of recurrent gastrointestinal bleeding in patients with cirrhosis, the use of prednisone for the treatment of those with severe alcoholic hepatitis, and the efficacy of liver transplantation in those with alcoholic cirrhosis.

Professor Poynard's work in viral hepatitis has made a

major contribution to our knowledge of the treatment of hepatitis B and C during the past decade. He is the author of four landmark papers published for the treatment of hepatitis C, namely a randomized trial of long-term treatments for chronic non-A and non-B hepatitis (1995), the natural history of liver fibrosis progression in patients with chronic hepatitis C (1997), a randomized trial of combination interferon-ribavirin for chronic hepatitis C (1998), and a prospective study of biochemical markers of liver fibrosis in chronic hepatitis C (2001).

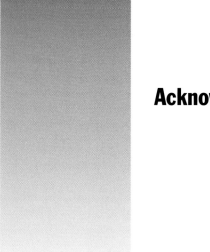

Acknowledgements

The author would like to thank the following:

Prof. Pierre Bedossa at l'Hôpital de Bicêtre; my colleagues in the Pitié-Salpêtrière, who are Prof. Pierre Opolon, Prof. Patrice Cacoub, Dr Yves Benhamou, Dr Brigitte Bernard, Dr Vlad Ratziu, Dr Vincent Di Martino, Dr Julien Taieb, Dr Joseph Moussalli, Dr Corinne Regimbeau, Dr Dominique Thabut, Dr Luminitza Bonihaye, Dr Mercedes de Torres, Dr Cecilia d'Arondel and Dr Marie Bochet; Dr Philippe Mathurin (Antoine Beclère Hospital, Clamart), Mrs Janice Albrecht (SPRI, Kenilworth, USA), Dr John Wong (Boston, USA), Dr John McHutchison (La Jolla, USA); Dan Edwards (London, UK).

Dedication

This book is dedicated to all members of our hepatitis team in the Service d'Hépato-Gastroentérologie at the Groupe Hospitalier Pitié-Salpêtrière in Paris (secretary, technicians, nurses and colleagues), and to Geneviève for her truffle forest in Eygalières.

Introduction

Chronic hepatitis B and C affect 520 million people worldwide.

Chronic hepatitis B virus infection is still a major cause of chronic liver disease and of mortality throughout the world, despite the efficacy of the vaccine. The natural history is better understood through greater knowledge of mutants and a spectacular increase in the sensitivity of viral load assessment. In recent years treatment has also been improved by the approval of lamivudine. This nucleoside has a very rapid efficacy in comparison to interferon and is better tolerated, but is associated with escape mutants.

Part I aims to present a contemporary approach to the natural history, the utility of serum markers and the management of chronic hepatitis B infection.

Chronic hepatitis C virus infection is a major cause of chronic liver disease with increasing mortality throughout the world. There is now very effective treatment enabling virus eradication in 60% of cases and reduction of progression to cirrhosis in the others. Therefore this infection should be largely detected and treated when necessary.

Part II aims to present a contemporary approach to the natural history and to the management of chronic hepatitis C virus infection. Many people infected have no specific symptoms and the treatment has several adverse events. Therefore the explanation to the patient of the disease as well as the explanation of the long-term treatment benefit is particularly important.

Hepatitis B

Natural history of hepatitis B: Epidemiology

1

Despite discovery of the virus more than 30 years ago,[1] the efficacy of hepatitis B virus (HBV) vaccine[2] and the advances in therapy (Figure 1.1) hepatitis B still remains an important public-health problem.

Prevalence

It has been estimated that 350 million people worldwide are chronic HBV carriers.[3] The global prevalence of chronic

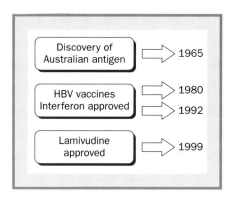

Figure 1.1
Landmarks in HBV therapy.

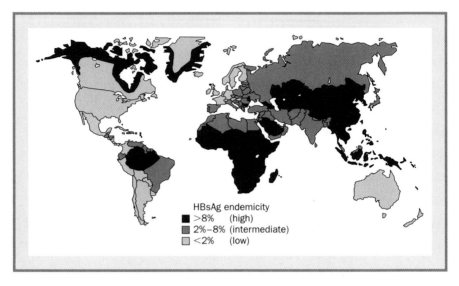

HBsAg endemicity
- >8% (high)
- 2%–8% (intermediate)
- <2% (low)

Figure 1.2
Worldwide prevalence of HBV in 1997.

HBV infection varies widely (Figure 1.2), from high (>8%, eg, in Africa, Asia, and the Western Pacific) to intermediate (2–7%, eg, in southern and eastern Europe) and low (<2%, eg, in western Europe, North America, and Australia).

These individuals are at risk of developing hepatological and non-hepatological manifestations. Between a third and a quarter of people infected chronically with HBV are expected to develop progressive liver disease (including cirrhosis and primary liver cancer).

Hepatitis B can cause cirrhosis, digestive haemorrhage, liver failure, and liver cancer.[3]

Serological markers and interpretation

Knowledge of the virus genome has allowed us to formulate several serological markers of HBV infection. The interpretation of HBV serological markers is described in Table 1.1.

In clinical practice chronic HBV carriers may be divided into two easily identifiable

Table 1.1 Interpretation of serological markers according to symptoms, transaminases, and histological features.

	HBsAg	HBsAb	HBeAg	HBeAb	Anti HBc-IgG	Anti HBc-IgM	HBV-DNA	Symptoms	ALT	Histological activity and fibrosis
Acute	+	–	+	+/–	+/–	+	+	+/–	++	++
Chronic carrier wild type	+	–	+	–	+	–	+	+/–	+/–	+/–+
Chronic carrier pre-core mutant*	+	–	–	+	+	–/+	+	+/–	+/–	+/–+
"Healthy carrier"†	+	–	–	+	+	–	–	–	–	–
"Immune-tolerance"†	+	–	+	–	+	–	++	–	–	–
Recovery/immunity	–	+	–	+	+	–	–	–	–	–
Immunity from vaccination	–	+	–	–	–	–	–	–	–	–
Occult infection‡	–	+/–	–	–	+/–	–	+/–	+/–	+/–	+/–+/–

*During flare-up antiHBc-IgM can be elevated; †Carrier without symptoms, normal transaminases, and with normal biopsy are divided into "healthy carriers" with undetectable HBV-DNA and patients with detectable HBV-DNA ("immune tolerance"). In these patients a risk of cirrhosis or hepatocellular carcinoma cannot be excluded. Pre-core mutant cannot be excluded. Pre-core mutant can be detected; ‡ HBV DNA can be detected in the liver in absence of serological markers.
ALT: Alanine aminotransferase.

serological types: those who are positive for HBeAg ("wild type") and those who are HBeAg negative and positive for anti-HBe.

HBV variants

The repression of the synthesis of wild-type HBV is because of defective variants with mutation in the core region. Among these variants, the most common in the Mediterranean area are mutants containing a strategic mutation at nucleotide 1896 of the pre-core region that prevents the secretion of HBeAg ("pre-core mutant").[4,5] HBeAg-negative, anti-HBe-positive chronic hepatitis B accounts for 7–30% of patients with chronic hepatitis worldwide. Prevalence rates range from 40–80% in the Mediterranean area, Hong-Kong, Korea, Taiwan and Japan to 13–15% in India and China to lower rates in northern Europe and the United States. The geographical variability in the prevalence of pre-core mutants may be related to the geographical variability of HBV genotype.

Most of variants seem to occur in the long-term natural history of wild type HBV but the exact prevalence of direct infection (transfusion, vertical or sexual) is unknown.[5–8] Several studies have documented progression from wild type to mutation 1896.[9–11]

HBV genotypes

Full-length sequence and phylogenetic analysis have isolated seven genotypes from A to G, the most prevalent in western countries being genotype A and D.[7] Subtypes are the variation of amino acids on the HBsAg. The four standards are adr, adw, ayw, and ayr. The most frequent combination of genotypes and subtypes are genotype A (subtype adw) in western Europe, D (subtype ayw) in the Mediterranean area, and G in France.

Genotype D and F of HBV tolerate the 1896 mutation whereas the mutation occurring within A and E genotypes generates non-viable mutants. The prevalence of genotype D matches the prevalence of pre-core mutants in the Mediterranean area. Mutation 1896 seems more frequent in genotype D than in genotype A.

Routes of transmission

The predominant routes of transmission vary according to the endemicity of the HBV infection. In areas of high endemicity, perinatal transmission is the main route of transmission, whereas in areas of low endemicity, sexual contact among high-risk adults is predominant (Table 1.2).[7,8]

Table 1.2 Risk groups for HBV infection among non-vaccinated people.

Areas of high HBV prevalence	*Vertical transmission: infants born to HBV-infected mothers.*
	Horizontal transmission within families (first 10 years).
Areas of intermediate HBV prevalence	*Horizontal transmission: older children, adolescents and adults.*
Areas of low prevalence	*High-risk sexual behaviour, multiple partners, HIV, genital herpes.*
	Intravenous drug users, even briefly and many years ago.
	Frequent exposure to blood products: haemophilia, transplants, haemodialysis, chronic renal failure, gammaglobulins, cancer chemotherapy.
	Health-care workers with needle-stick accidents.
	Blood transfusion before 1970.

Natural history of hepatitis B: Hepatic manifestations

2

The major hepatological consequences of HBV infection is the progression to cirrhosis and its potential complications: haemorrhage, hepatic insufficiency, and primary liver cancer (Table 2.1).

Contrary to HCV infection, current understanding of the natural history of HBV (Figure 2.1) infection has not been well analysed by assessment of liver-fibrosis progression. The clinical and histological outcome of chronic HBV infection is closely related to the pathobiology of the virus and the host immune response.

Virus genotype, persistence and strength of replication, emergence of viral mutants or integration of viral genomic material into the hepatocyte genome play a part in the natural history. So far these factors have not been clearly assessed.[7,8] The age at infection is most often unknown in patients without vertical transmission; the sensitivity of HBV-DNA assays are improving every year.

HBV is in general not a cytopathic virus. In most patients with chronic hepatitis B, there is no direct correlation between the viral load and the severity of liver disease.

Table 2.1 Natural history of HBV carriers.

First author	Number of patients	Age at baseline	Duration of Follow-up	Evolution	Liver complications	Death related to liver
Bortolotti	185	<10 years	13 years	5% became HBsAg negative 7% still HBe positive	2 hepatocellular carcinoma	
HBeAg positive baseline	168			83% became anti-HBe and asymptomatic		
HBeAg negative baseline	17			3% reactivation 2% elevated transaminases and anti-HBe		
MacMahon	1400	46 years	5 years	No vasculitis, no cryoglobulinaemia	14 chronic active hepatitis 8 cirrhosis 20 hepatocellular carcinoma	13 hepatocellular carcinoma
Sakuma	202	45 years	5 years	9% persistent abnormal transaminases 76% persistent normal transaminases	5 hepatocellular carcinoma (4 cirrhosis)	4 hepatocellular carcinoma (3 had normal transaminases at baseline)

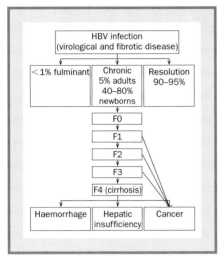

Figure 2.1
Natural history of HBV virus infection. Estimated key numbers of HBV natural history from literature and our database: median time from infection (F0) to cirrhosis (F4) is 30 years. Mortality at 10 years for cirrhosis is 50%. Transition probability per year from non-complicated cirrhosis to each of the complications is around 3%. Less than 10% of cancer occurred in non-cirrhotic liver.

Can a healthy carrier state be defined?

Most longitudinal or cross-sectional studies in HBV have separated a so-called "healthy" carrier state, a phase of chronic hepatitis and cirrhosis. The definition of "healthy HBV carrier" is not clear and therefore could be dangerous for patients. If the definition is the absence of symptoms, the absence of transaminases elevation, and the absence of abnormalities in the liver (inflammation, necrosis or fibrosis), these negative findings should have been observed at least twice. This is not the case in the published cohorts (Figure 2.2). Despite a good overall prognosis[12,13] the status of "healthy HBV carrier" is not definitive and some patients can progress to cirrhosis and/or to hepatocellular carcinoma (Table 2.2).[14–16] We observed significant fibrosis (septal fibrosis or cirrhosis)

Table 2.2 Natural history of "healthy carriers".

First author	Number of patients	Age at follow-up	Duration of follow-up	Liver complications	Death related to liver	HBsAg negativation rate per year
Villeneuve	317	46 years	16 years	0 liver cancer	4 cirrhosis	0.7%
de Franchis	92		10 years	1 cirrhosis	0	15%
				0 liver cancer		

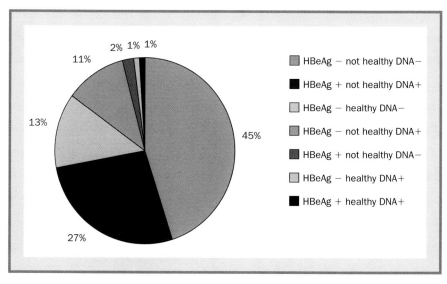

Figure 2.2
Prevalence of HBeAg and detectable HBV-DNA in a cohort of 223 patients HBsAg positive. 70% were HBeAg negative, 15% were healthy carrier (absence of symptoms, normal transaminases, and absence of necrosis, inflammation, and fibrosis at liver biopsy [AOFO]; among these healthy carriers only four had detectable HBV DNA).

in 30% of 163 HBsAg positive patients with undetectable serum HBV-DNA.[17,18] Even in patients with disappearance of hepatitis B surface antigen and presence of anti-HBs, liver complications may occur.[19]

Clinical significance of HBV variants

Few cross sectional or longitudinal studies have compared the clinical importance of chronic HBV carriers who are positive for HBeAg ("wild type") and those who are HBeAg negative and positive for anti-HBe (Table 2.3).[6,15–22] HBeAg negative patients were older which may explain the higher prevalence of fibrosis.

Very few patients have been followed longitudinally with virologic assessment.[20] Among 12 HBeAg-positive patients with chronic hepatitis, who seroconverted to anti-HBe during follow-up, anti-HBe seroconversion was accompanied by a dramatic reduction of HBV replication and

Table 2.3 Comparison between HBV carriers with HBeAg positive versus anti-HBe positive.

First author	Number of patients	Age (years) at biopsy	Male	Asian or African origin	HBV DNA detectable	Normal transaminases	Significant fibrosis (F2/F3/F4)	Cirrhosis	Significant activity (A2/A3)
Poynard									
HBeAg positive	491	35	74%	62%	100%	14%	22%	7%	50%
HBeAg negative	286	41	76%	43%	39%	43%	42%	15%	23%
HBV-DNApos	113	44	80%	17%	100%	11%	57%	21%	43%
HBV-DNAneg	173	40	73%	79%	0%	54%	32%	11%	19%
Zarski									
HBeAg positive	215	36	83%	17%	100%	100%		17%	
HBeAg negative	61	44	84%	26%	100%	100%		38%	

normalization of transaminases in all except one, and by the emergence of pre-core mutant (1896 point mutation) that replaced the wild type in seven of the 12. Of the seven who harboured the pre-core mutant, three continued to show normal transaminases during subsequent follow-up, three had mild transaminases elevation, and one had an acute short-lived reactivation after 4 years of normal transaminases. The five cases that continued to show prevalence of wild type in spite of anti-HBe seroconversion all revealed persistently normal transaminases.

Association with hepatocellular carcinoma

An association between HBV infection and occurrence of primary liver cancer (hepatocellular carcinoma) was observed soon after the discovery of HBV and largely confirmed thereafter.[23–27]

These lines of evidence were based on epidemiological associations in areas of high prevalence,[25] on molecular studies in hepatocellular carcinoma cell lines,[26] and on animal models.[27] In endemic areas such as China and sub-Saharian Africa, where the HBsAg carrier rate is 10%, primary liver cancer presents an incidence of up to 150 cases per 100 000 per year. By contrast, in the United States, where the carrier rate is less than 1%, the incidence of primary liver cancer

is four cases per 100 000 per year. The prevalence of HBsAg among patients with primary liver cancer varies from 85–95% in Africa and Asia to 10–25% in western Europe and the United States.[28] A further support for this association was the decrease in childhood primary liver cancer after the implementation of a universal vaccination programme for newborns.[29] The incidence of liver cancer among HBV carriers is associated with the duration of infection, male sex, and the length and severity of liver disease (Figure 2.3).[30]

Occult infection

HBV DNA can be detected in the liver of patients without HBsAg detectable in the

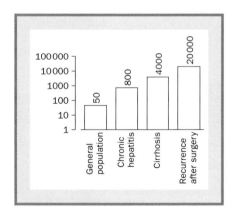

Figure 2.3
Annual incidence (cases per 100 000) of hepatocellular carcinoma according to the stage of liver disease. Adapted with permission.[30]

Table 2.4 *Factors associated with progression to cirrhosis or to cancer in HBV carriers*

Factors	Cirrhosis	Hepatocellular carcinoma
Age at infection	Yes	Yes
Duration of infection	Yes	Yes
Male sex	Yes	Yes
Age at biopsy	Yes	Yes
Consumption of alcohol >50 g per day	Yes	Yes
HCV coinfection	Yes	Not sure
Delta coinfection	Yes	Not sure
CD4 count <200/mL	Yes	Not sure
Fibrosis stage	Yes	Yes
Necrosis	Not sure	Not sure
Inflammation	Not sure	Not sure
Genotype	Not sure	Not sure
Pre-core mutant	Not sure	Not sure
Core-promoter mutant	Not sure	Not sure
Seroconversion anti-HBe	Not sure	Not sure
HBV-DNA level	Not sure	Not sure
Aflatoxin	Not sure	Yes

serum.[31] The lack of HBsAg may be due to rearrangements in the HBV genome that interfere with gene expression or lead to the production of an antigenically modified S protein.[32] Clearance of serum HBsAg may also occur without clearance of HBV DNA in the liver.[33]

Factors associated with fibrosis progression

There is little information concerning the annual rate of development of cirrhosis in chronic HBV carriers as well as risk factors associated with the fibrosis progression rate. Factors associated and not associated with cirrhosis or hepatocellular carcinoma are summarized in Table 2.4.[3,7,8]

Natural history of hepatitis B: Extra-hepatic manifestations and quality of life

3

Extra-hepatic manifestation

Since the recognition of HBV,[34] many extrahepatic manifestations have been reported with HBV infection including vasculitis (polyarteritis nodosa), glomerulonephritis, mixed cryoglobulinemia, skin rash, arthritis, arthralgia, and papular acrodermatitis (Table 3.1).[34–41]

Table 3.1 Extrahepatic manifestations in HBV.

Chronic hepatitis
Polyarteritis nodosa
Glomerulonephritis
   Membranous
    Mesangial proliferative
    Membranoproliferative
Cryoglobulinaemia

Acute hepatitis
Arthralgia
Arthritis
Skin rashes
Serum sickness-like manifestations
Urticaria
Papular acrodermatitis

Vasculitis

Systemic vasculitis (systemic necrotizing vasculitis or polyarteritis nodosa [PAN]), is the most severe symptomatic extra-hepatic manifestation, although rare (1%). 30–70% of patients with PAN are infected with HBV. The initial illness presents with abdominal pain, fever, rash, polyarthralgias, polyarthritis, hypertension, and eosinophilia; it can progress to multisystem vasculitis involving the kidneys, gastrointestinal tract, peripheral and central nervous system. Medium to small arteries are involved by fibrinoid necrosis and perivascular infiltration. Angiographic findings include microaneurysms, stenosis, and occlusion of arteries mainly in the kidney, liver, and intestine. The mortality rate is high (30–50%) and not associated with the hepatitis severity.

Glomerulonephritis

Most of the patients have the nephrotic syndrome with an 85% rate of spontaneous remission after 2 years. Despite the limited number of studies the benign natural history seems more frequent in children than in adults. Membranous glomerulonephritis is the most common pathological finding, especially in children, and is usually associated with capillary wall deposits of HBeAg. Membrano-proliferative glomerulonephritis is less frequent, more often described in adults and associated with capillary wall deposits of HBsAg. Such glomerulonephritis seems to result from immune complex-mediated injury but factors to explain why only few patients experience this injury are unknown.[40]

Cryoglobulin

The strong association observed between mixed cryoglobulinaemia and chronic HBV was in retrospect mostly related to hepatitis C coinfection.[41] The prevalence of cryoglobulin-positive patients in hepatitis B is three times lower than in hepatitis C. Cryoglobulin-positive patients have mixed type II cryoglobulins or type III.

Health-related quality of life

One way to assess the clinical impact of hepatic and extra-hepatic manifestation among patients infected by HBV is to assess the health-related quality of life. Patients with chronic HBV infection showed a reduction in the SF36 scores that assessed mental functions, but they had no decrease in the scores that measured physical symptoms.[42,43]

Median utilities for mildly symptomatic HBV infection and severely symptomatic HBV infection are significantly decreased in comparison with asymptomatic HBV infection. For severely symptomatic HBV infection there was no difference in comparison with the quality of life of patients with AIDS (Figure 3.1).[43]

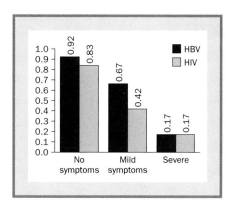

Figure 3.1
Quality of life impaired among patients infected with hepatitis B. 0 = death; 1 = good health. Median utilities estimated by 200 housestaff and staff physicians infected by HBV or HIV according to three stages. For HIV severe infection was AIDS. All differences versus asymptomatic stage were significant (p < 0.01 or each two-way comparison). There was no difference between the two severe stages. Adapted with permission.[43]

4

Goal of treatment in chronic hepatitis B

The optimal goal is to eliminate the virus completely and permanently. In fact, as with hepatitis C, there is nowadays two separate goals: the first goal is to achieve a sustained clearance of the virus; the second goal in patients without a sustained virological response is to reduce the liver injury (reduce fibrosis progression in non-cirrhotic patients), to prevent cirrhosis complications, to improve quality of life, and to reduce infectivity (Table 4.1).

Table 4.1 Endpoints of treatment in chronic hepatitis B.

Endpoints	Optimal goal	Suppressive goal
Seroconversion in HBsAg	Yes	No
Seroconversion in HBeAg for wild type	Yes	No
Serum HBV-DNA undetectable*	Yes	No
Normalization of transaminase activity	Yes	No
Disappearance of liver fibrosis	Yes	No
Disappearance of necrosis and inflammation	Yes	No
Reduction of fibrosis progression	Yes	Yes
Reduction of necrosis and inflammation	Yes	Yes
Improvement of quality of life	Yes	Yes
Reduction of infectivity	Yes	Yes
Reduction of morbidity	Yes	Yes
Reduction of mortality	Yes	Yes

*HBV-DNA detection methods have a large range of sensitivity from 1000 (PCR assay) to 1 million copies per mL

Efficacy of interferon

5

Biological effect

Interferon-alfa was the first drug approved for the treatment of chronic hepatitis B in 1992 in the United States and Europe. Interferon-alfa binds to specific cell receptors and produces immunomodulatory, antiviral, and antifibrotic effects (Table 5.1). Interferon increases activity of macrophages, natural killer cells, and cytotoxic T cells, which

Table 5.1 Different effects of interferon-alfa.

Antiviral effect	Immunomodulatory	Anti-fibrotic
Increases macrophage activity	Increases Th1 effect (interleukin 12)	Reduces stellate cell activation
Increases natural killer cell activity	Increases HLA I expression	Activates collagenases
Increases cytotoxic T cell activity	Increases B cell proliferation	
Activates 2-5-oligoanenylate synthetase, which reduces viral RNA Activates Protein kinase P1, which reduces viral protein synthesis	Modulates Th2 effect	

mediate the elimination of virus-infected cells. Antiviral properties of interferon-alfa include inhibition of virus entry into cells and the reduction viral RNA and protein synthesis.

Clinical effect

Interferon-alfa in doses of at least 5 million three times a week has been shown to induce virological and biological responses in 30–50% of treated patients in comparison with a spontaneous remission rate of 5–15% in controls (Figure 5.1).[44,45] The recommended regimen of interferon-alfa is either 5 million units daily or 10 million units thrice weekly, subcutaneously for 4 months.[44] Liver biopsy at 6 months or more after

completion of treatment shows improvement in necrosis and inflammation.[46] Extrahepatic manifestations of infection have also demonstrated a response to interferon.[35]

Durability of response and long-term outcome

Interferon-alfa-induced HBeAg clearance has been reported to be durable in 80–90% of patients after a follow-up of 4–8 years.[44]

Data on long-term outcome of interferon-treated patients are limited. Patients who cleared HBeAg had better rates of survival and survival free of hepatic decompensation (Figures 5.2 and 5.3).[47,48]

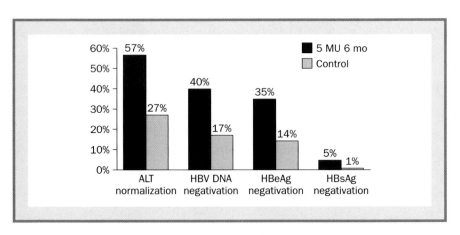

Figure 5.1
Meta-analysis of 15 randomized trials to compare interferon with control in patients with chronic hepatitis B. Adapted with permission.[45]

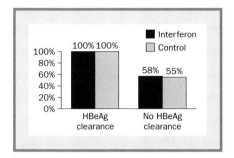

Figure 5.2
Long-term efficacy of interferon: 8 years survival and HBeAg status. Adapted with permission.[47]

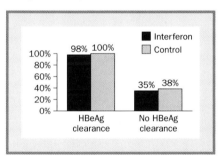

Figure 5.3
Long-term efficacy of interferon: 8 years survival without complications and HBeAg status. Adapted with permission.[47]

Predictive factors of response

Seven factors are associated with a sustained beneficial response to interferon (Table 5.2). The most important are high transaminases and low serum HBV DNA, which are probably indirect markers of endogenous

immune clearance.[8,44] When adjusted on transaminases and HBV DNA the response rates are similar between Asian and white patients.[8]

Patients HBeAg positive, HBV DNA positive, and with persistently normal ALT are usually children or young adults with perinatally acquired HBV infection. The response rate for interferon is low, lower than 10%, and the benefit risk is not known.[8] However, the long-term benefit in terms of reduction of fibrosis progression has not been assessed.

In patients with compensated cirrhosis interferon is safe and may be effective. In patients with decompensated cirrhosis interferon is not contraindicated but sepsis and exacerbation of liver disease have been described.[49]

Table 5.2 Factors associated with sustained beneficial response to interferon-alfa in patients with chronic hepatitis B.

Beneficial factors
Short duration of disease
High serum transaminases activity
Low serum HBV DNA level
Active histological changes (inflammation and necrosis)
Wild type (HBeAg positive) virus
Absence of decompensated cirrhosis
Absence of immunosuppression

Efficacy of lamivudine

6

Lamivudine is the (-) enantiomer of 2'3' dideoxy-3'-thiacytidine. It is phosphorylated to the triphosphate, which competes with the other triphosphates for incorporation into DNA, causing chain termination. By decreasing viral load lamivudine may also reverse the T-cell hyporesponsiveness to hepatitis B viral antigens.

Efficacy has been observed first among patients coinfected by HIV and HBV.[50–52] Several randomized clinical trials have shown the efficacy of lamivudine 100 mg per day in immunocompetent patients infected by wild type[53–55] or precore[56] HBV (Figure 6.1).

1 year efficacy in patients infected with wild type HBV (HBeAg positive)

During 52 weeks of treatment lamivudine is effective in comparison with placebo on almost all endpoints: transaminases, HBV DNA measured by non-PCR-methods, HBe seroconversion, necrosis, inflammation, and fibrosis. There was no difference for HBsAg (Figures 6.2 and 6.3).

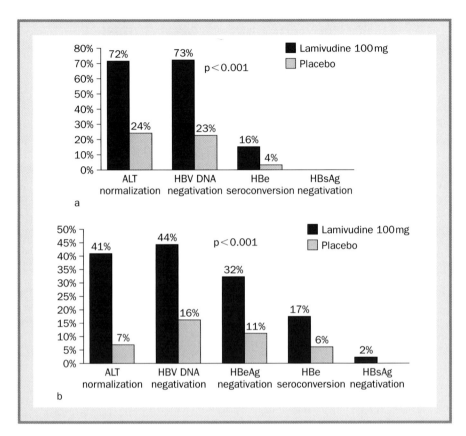

Figure 6.1
Efficacy of 52 weeks lamivudine on transaminases and virological endpoints. a) Chinese trial. b) US trial.
Adapted with permission.[54,55]

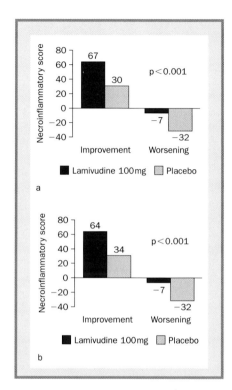

Figure 6.2
Efficacy (% of patients) of 42 weeks lamivudine on necrosis and inflammation in wild-type HBV. a) Chinese trial. b) US trial. Adapted with permission.[54,55]

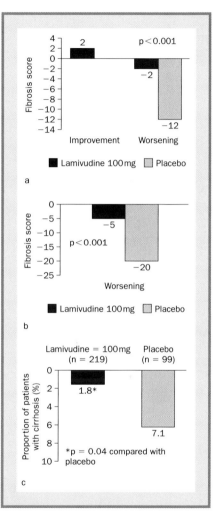

Figure 6.3
Efficacy of lamivudine on fibrosis progression in wild-type HBV. a) Chinese trial. b) US trial. Adapted with permission.[54,55] c) Combination of individual data from lamivudine trials.[63] Adapted with permission of Glaxo-Wellcome.

Efficacy in patients infected with pre-core mutant HBV (HBeAg negative)

There are fewer trials in pre-core HBV infection. In one randomized trial lamivudine was effective at 24 weeks versus placebo[56] on transaminases and HBV-DNA (Figure 6.4). Biopsy samples were not taken in the control group and results after 48 weeks of treatment were not controlled. However, there was a similar effect compared to that observed in wild type on necrosis, inflammation, and fibrosis worsening (Figure 6.4).

Predictive factors of response

Some factors are associated with a beneficial response to lamivudine rather than interferon (Table 6.1). However, there are differences in comparison with interferon because

Table 6.1 Factors associated with beneficial response to lamivudine in patients with chronic hepatitis B.

Beneficial factors
High-serum transaminases activity Low-serum HBV DNA level Wild-type (HBeAg positive) virus? Absence of immunosuppression?

lamivudine seems just as effective in patients with immunosuppression as patients coinfected with HIV[50–52] or transplanted patients.[57] The biggest difference probably concerns the treatment of patients with decompensated cirrhosis. Lamivudine is very effective with a rapid clinical improvement (Figure 6.5).[58]

Efficacy of lamivudine after 1 year of treatment: incidence of YMDD mutant HBV

After 1 year the benefit:risk ratio of lamivudine is more difficult to assess because the long-term treatment of lamivudine is associated with a higher response rate, defined as HBeAg seroconversion,[59] and also with a linear increase of escape mutant called YMDD.[52,60,61] In a small non-randomized cohort the seroconversion rate was 40% at 4 years (Figure 6.6).[59]

Preliminary data suggest that there is a durability of response (HBeAg negative) in more than 80% of 43 patients with a 21 month median follow-up (Schiff E EASL meeting, 2000). Because of the high relapse rate after 8 months treatment of at least 48 weeks is recommended.

Lamivudine resistant mutants

Selection of lamivudine-resistant mutants is a main concern; the most common mutation

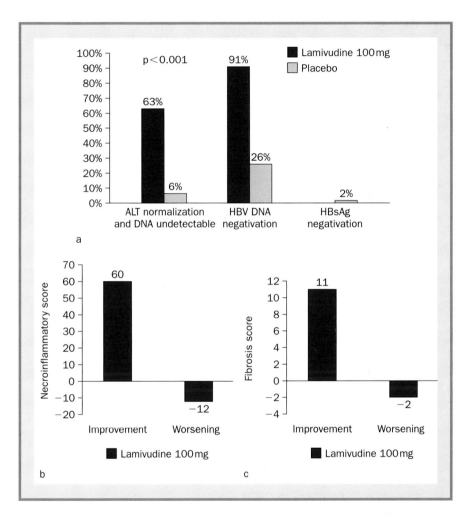

Figure 6.4
*Efficacy of lamivudine on transaminases, and virological and histological endpoints in pre-core mutant HBV.
a) Transaminases, HBV DNA, and HBeAg (24 weeks). b) Necrosis and inflammation (42 weeks). c) Fibrosis
(42 weeks). Adapted with permission.[56]*

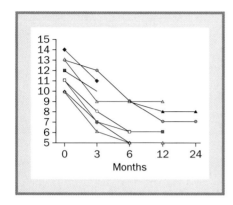

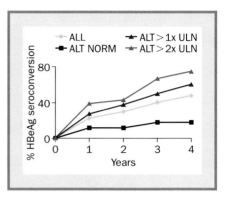

Figure 6.5
Efficacy of lamivudine 100 mg in 13 severely decompensated cirrhotic patients. Adapted with permission.[58]

Figure 6.6
4 years lamivudine treatment of wild-type HBV. Adapted with permission.[59]

affects the YMDD motif of the HBV DNA polymerase. The development of resistance is easily shown by a reappearance of HBV DNA in the serum after an initial disappearance in the absence of non-compliance. The incidence is around 15% a year.[51,59–61] An increased risk of lamivudine resistance has been suggested in HBV subtype adw in a few patients and this has to be confirmed.[62]

The clinical course of patients with lamivudine-resistant mutant is usually better than in non-treated patients. In rare cases emergence of mutants may be associated with acute exacerbations of liver disease or hepatic decompensation. However, most patients who continue treatment have lower serum HBV DNA and transaminase levels compared with pre-treatment (Figure 6.7). HBeAg seroconversion has been reported in 25% of patients who continued lamivudine after detection of mutants.[59]

Cessation of treatment in patients with severe liver disease is a major concern as a flare-up of liver disease is possible as well as liver failure, due to an uncontrolled replication of wild-type HBV.[60] In patients with severe disease it is therefore recommended to continue lamivudine and to use new drugs effective on YMDD mutant, such as adefovir or entecavir (compassionate programme or randomized trial).

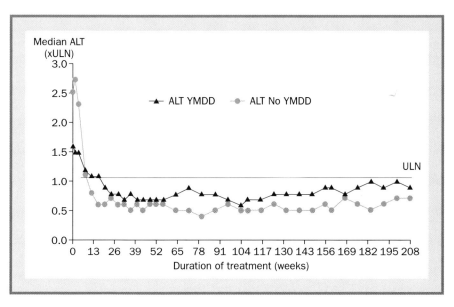

Figure 6.7
4 years follow-up of patients treated with lamivudine 100 mg according to the presence (n = 39) or absence (n = 19) of YMDD mutant. Adapted with permission.[59]

When to stop lamivudine?

In wild-type HBV lamivudine can be stopped when there is a HBeAg seroconversion with detectable HBeAb, undetectable HBV-DNA, and normal transaminases. At least 1 year of treatment is recommended.

In pre-core mutant HBV lamivudine can be stopped when transaminases are normal and HBV-DNA undetectable. It is not clear but at least 1 year of treatment is recommended as well as at least 1 month with undetectable HBV-DNA and normal ALT.

Comparison between lamivudine, interferon, and combination interferon lamivudine

7

Only one published randomized trial has compared
lamivudine 100 mg monotherapy 48 weeks versus interferon
(16 weeks) and versus combination interferon lamivudine
(24 weeks). A total of 226 patients were included.[63] There was
no significant difference between the arms of the trial for
the virological and histological endpoints (Figure 7.1).
Contrary to what was expected there was also no significant
difference between regimen in the flare-up incidences after
the end of treatment (Figure 7.2).

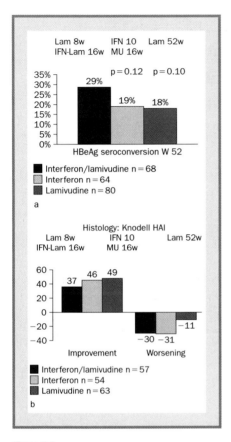

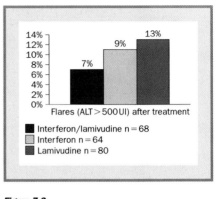

Figure 7.2
Comparison between lamivudine, interferon, and interferon/lamivudine combination for flare-ups after the end of treatment. Adapted with permission.[63]

Figure 7.1
Comparison between lamivudine, interferon, and interferon/lamivudine combination for HBeAg seroconversion and necrosis and inflammation. a) HBeAg seroconversion. b) Necrosis and inflammation. Adapted with permission.[63]

Safety of lamivudine

8

Lamivudine is in general very well tolerated, with similar occurrence of clinical and biological adverse events in patients receiving lamivudine or placebo.

As observed by 4 years follow-up, 15% occurrence per year of YMDD mutant was not associated with severe adverse events (Table 8.1).

The safety of interferon is discussed in the hepatitis C section.

Table 8.1 Serious adverse events in each year. Safety database, adapted with permission from GlaxoWellcome.

Therapy	Year of therapy	Number of patients	Patients with severe adverse events	Liver-disease related
Placebo	1	200	17 (8.5%)	4 (2.0%)
Lamivudine 100 mg	1	999	42 (4.2%)	7 (0.7%)
Lamivudine 100 mg	2	741	24 (3.2%)	15 (2.0%)
Lamivudine 100 mg	3	630	26 (4.1%)	12 (1.9%)
Lamivudine 100 mg	4	208	8 (3.8%)	3 (1.4%)

New drugs effective on YMDD mutant

9

Adefovir dipivoxil has potent *in vivo* and *in vitro* activity against both wild-type and lamivudine-resistant HBV.[64–67] We evaluated the safety and efficacy of adefovir dipivoxil 10 mg once daily in the treatment of lamivudine-resistant HBV infection in 35 HIV-infected patients in an open-label trial.[68] Mean decrease in HBV DNA serum levels from baseline (8.64 ± 0.08 $\log_{10}$ copies/mL) was -2.90 ± 0.11 $\log_{10}$ copies/mL and -3.40 ± 0.14 $\log_{10}$ copies/mL at week 24 ($p < 0.0001$); (Figure 9.1). Adefovir was generally well tolerated. Entecavir is also in phase III trials with a possible efficacy in YMDD mutant.[69]

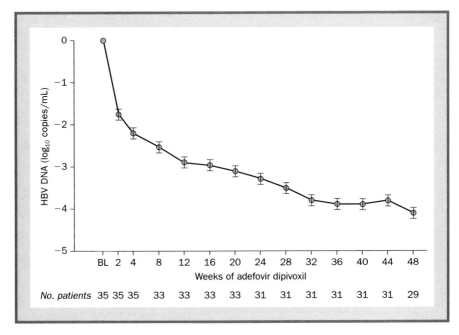

Figure 9.1
Mean changes from baseline in serum HBV DNA measured by PCR during adefovir dipivoxil therapy in HIV/HBV coinfected patients. Adapted with permission.[68]

First-line treatment of chronic hepatitis B: lamivudine or interferon?

10

There is no clear consensus except that lamivudine in patients with cirrhosis is best with contraindications to interferon.

In naïve patients there is a choice between lamivudine and interferon according to their advantages and disadvantages (Table 10.1).

One possibility is to start with lamivudine and to switch to interferon if resistant mutant occurs. The development of adefovir and entecavir are also reassuring for the management of resistant mutant. Combination therapy with lamivudine, PEG-interferon, adefovir, and entecavir are needed to improve treatment of chronic hepatitis B both for wild-type (Figure 10.1) and pre-core mutant (Figure 10.2).

Table 10.1 Advantages and disadvantages of lamivudine and interferon.

Advantages	Disadvantages
Lamivudine	
• Oral administration	• Long duration of therapy
• Minimal adverse events	• Resistant mutants
• Useful in decompensated cirrhosis	• Durability of response?
• Useful in post-transplantation	
• Fast efficacy on transaminases and HBV-DNA	
Interferon	
• Short course: 16–24 weeks	• Many "problem" patients
• No drug-resistant mutants	• Significant adverse events
• Well-established track record	

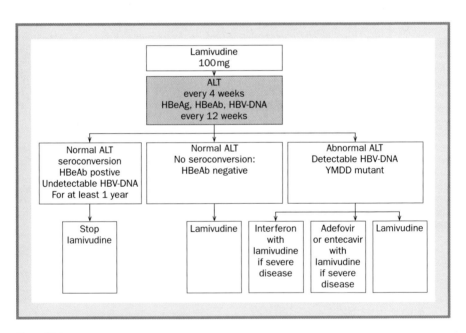

Figure 10.1
Recommendation for wild-type HBV chronic hepatitis management.

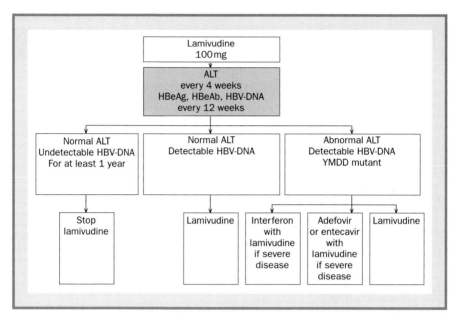

Figure 10.2
Recommendation for pre-core mutant HBV chronic hepatitis management.

Who needs to be treated and how to explain the goals to the patient

11

Given the natural history of hepatitis B there are four different goals for treatment: 1) To prevent the occurrence of cirrhosis and its complications. 2) To prevent occurrence of hepatocellular carcinoma possible even in the absence of cirrhosis. 3) To reduce the extrahepatic manifestations. 4) To prevent the contamination of other people (ie, surgeon or drug user). Vaccination of relatives is mandatory.

Who needs to be treated

There is no clear consensus on who should be treated. Some experts recommend no treatment for patients with compensated liver disease with normal transaminases and for patients infected with pre-core mutant.[70]

Another recommendation is to perform liver biopsy in all patients with detectable HBV-DNA. If there is significant fibrosis or activity (necrosis and inflammation), and because of the risk of progression to cirrhosis, treatment is recommended.

If the patient is not at risk of developing cirrhosis, has no symptoms, and is not at risk of transmitting the virus there is

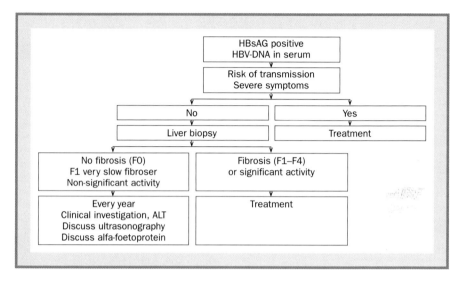

Figure 11.1
Treatment decisions in chronic hepatitis B.

no need to treat even if HBV-DNA is detectable (ie, 60-year-old asymptomatic patient contaminated after birth and without fibrosis at biopsy).

Patients with HBV-DNA detectable and with symptoms, or at risk of transmission (infectivity), or with an active cirrhosis should be treated.

One algorithm is suggested in Figure 11.1.

Ten key points for understanding the natural history of HBV

1. Almost all the mortality of the disease is related to complications of cirrhosis.
2. Rare cases of primary liver cancer can occur in the absence of cirrhosis.
3. One third of infected patients will probably never progress to cirrhosis or to cancer.
4. Definition of healthy carrier (normal transaminases, normal histology, no symptoms) is time dependent and a follow-up is highly recommended.

5. Despite the risk of fibrosis a patient can be treated for extra-hepatic manifestation or to prevent transmission of the virus.

6. Cryoglobulinaemia is observed in 10% of cases and rarely associated with severe symptoms (1% of vasculitis).

7. Viral load, serotype, and genotype are not related to severity of the disease.

8. Alcohol consumption greater than four glasses a day accelerates the fibrosis progression.

9. Normal transaminases do not exclude the presence of cirrhosis.

10. Relatives can be protected by vaccination.

Ten key points for understanding HBV treatment

1. There are two goals for the treatment of hepatic manifestation: the first goal is to eradicate the virus; if the virus is not eradicated the second goal is to prevent progression to cirrhosis, the complications of cirrhosis, and occurrence of primary liver cancer.

2. In wild-type HBV infection (HBeAg positive) the viral response is well defined by undetectable HBV-DNA, normal transaminases, undetectable HBeAg, and occurrence of HBeAb (seroconversion HBe).

3. In pre-core mutant HBV infection (HBeAg negative) the viral response is defined by undetectable HBV-DNA and normal transaminases.

4. Seroconversion of HBsAg (undetectable HBsAg and occurrence of HBsAb) occurs rarely after treatment.

5. When a sustained viral response is obtained there is a dramatic improvement of liver histology including necroinflammatory features in all patients and fibrosis stage in non-cirrhotic patients.

6. When a sustained viral response is obtained in cirrhotic patients, there is a major clinical improvement.

7. Occurrence of lamivudine-resistant mutant is the main concern of this regimen but a seroconversion can be obtained as well as lower HBV-DNA and transaminases in comparison with pretreatment values.

8. Depression and suicide are the most extreme adverse events of interferon.

9. New drugs effective on lamivudine-resistant mutant are in phase III trials.

10. Liver transplantation is no longer contraindicated in patients with HBV cirrhosis.

Management of relapsers and non-responders

12

Relapsers and non-responders to interferon should be treated by lamivudine. For relapsers and non-responders to lamivudine, interferon could be considered. In relapsers to lamivudine without resistant mutant a longer duration of lamivudine should be considered. Non-responders are most often patients with resistant mutant. If there is no severe liver disease lamivudine can be stopped and interferon started. If there is a severe liver disease (cirrhosis) there is a risk of decompensation. Adefovir or entecavir should be considered.

Management of patients coinfected by HBV and HIV

13

Among patients infected by HIV, HBV coinfection must be systematically screened and treatment of HBV must be discussed when fibrosis is observed at liver biopsy. When transaminase activity is increased in a patient infected by HIV with negative HCV PCR a serum HBV PCR must be administered because false negative HBsAg is possible in immunodepressed patients.

Most often patients coinfected by HBV and HIV are treated with anti-HIV treatment, including lamivudine. Lamivudine 100 mg monotherapy must not be given to patients infected by HIV because this dose is ineffective for HIV (300 mg is recommended) and without combined anti-HIV treatment there is a rapid risk of lamivudine-resistant mutant to HIV.

Lamivudine-resistant-mutant incidence is similar (15% per year) in HIV patients treated with anti-HIV combination in comparison with patients infected by HBV only.[52] Adefovir 10 mg per day is effective for the treatment of lamivudine-resistant mutant.[68]

Anti-HIV treatment is often associated with transaminases increase (D4T, DDI, abacavir, nevirapine, protease inhibitor). When the increase is important another liver biopsy must be discussed and compared with biopsy before treatment. The following factors can be involved: alcohol consumption, illicit intravenous drug injection, substitution drug toxicity, anti-HIV drug toxicity, coinfection with HCV, HBV or Delta virus, liver opportunistic infection, immune restoration, and sclerosing cholangitis. The impact of immune reconstitution on liver-fibrosis progression is unknown.

Management of transplanted patients infected by HBV

14

End-stage HBsAg-positive cirrhosis is one of the main indications for orthotopic liver transplantation. Recurrence of HBV infection is the most significant problem with an 85% rate in the absence of any prophylaxis. During the past 10 years substantial progress has been made with the passive prophylaxis with hepatitis B immunoglobulin (HBIg),[71] with the approval of lamivudine and the development of new potent antiviral agents.[71–74] The best algorithm is to obtain HBV DNA undetectable before transplantation. After transplantation combination of low-dose HBIg with lamivudine seems so far the best prophylaxis regimen. New nucleosides active on lamivudine resistant mutant (ie, adefovir, entecavir) are presently under investigation.

Cost-effectiveness of treatment

15

There were reductions in lifetime risk of developing compensated cirrhosis, decompensated cirrhosis, and hepatocellular carcinoma of 5%, 11%, and 11%, respectively, when lamivudine was available in comparison with interferon.[75] The introduction of lamivudine is expected to reduce and delay the progression of chronic hepatitis B, increasing life expectancy and quality of life of patients for a small overall increase in healthcare costs in comparison with interferon monotherapy (Tables 15.1 and 15.2).

Hepatitis C treatment in a patient coinfected by HIV and HBV

- If the patient is not treated for HIV and there is no indication for this treatment (rare event): a treatment by interferon monotherapy can be discussed if there is an extensive fibrosis or a minimal fibrosis with significant activity. If patient has a contraindication to interferon and a severe liver disease lamivudine should be recommended at 300 mg in combination with other anti HIV treatments.

- If the patient is not yet treated for HIV and there is an indication for this treatment: the treatment of HIV must be given including lamivudine at 300 mg.
- If the HBV infection is discovered when the patient is already under treatment for HIV, lamivudine 300 mg should be incorporated in the combination therapy.
- Alcohol consumption should be prohibited in all coinfected HIV-HBV patients because of the rapid progression from fibrosis to cirrhosis.

Table 15.1 Direct medical cost of HBV treatment for 1 year model. Values in parentheses indicate the values for patients who had seroconverted by the second 6 months. Adapted with permission.[75]

Cost	Cost per patient for one year (Australian $)		
	Lamivudine	Interferon	No treatment
Outpatient setting	200 (172)	591 (562)	200 (172)
Specialist room	281 (240)	216 (176)	281 (240)
Test/pathology	872 (782)	1144 (1054)	872 (782)
Drug	1376	3729	0
Total	2729 (2569)	5682 (5523)	1353 (1194)

Table 15.2 Cost-effectiveness of lamivudine therapy versus interferon. Adapted with permission.[75]

	Lamivudine regimen vs interferon regimen
Life expectancy	
Life expectancy years	3.9 years increase
Quality-adjusted life years	3.2 years increase
Incremental cost	
Per life year	633 Australian $ increase
Per quality-adjusted life year	735 Australian $ increase

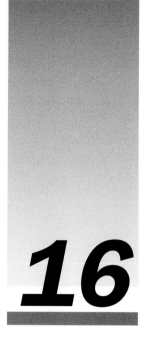

Practical guidelines for the management of hepatitis B

Liver biopsy

HBsAg and HBV-DNA detection serum testing is essential for the diagnosis of hepatitis B infection. However, biopsy is necessary for staging the severity of disease (fibrosis stage) and grading the amount of necrosis and inflammation. Biopsy is also helpful in ruling out other causes of liver disease such as alcoholic features, non-alcoholic steato-hepatitis, autoimmune hepatitis, medication-induced, coinfection with HCV, HIV, or iron overload.

Liver biopsy is helpful before treating a patient, for the decision and the duration of therapy. Biopsy is usually not helpful when cirrhosis is clinically or biologically obvious.

Liver biopsy is usually done by intercostal route. In case of clotting disorders transjugular route is used.

HBV-DNA detection

PCR can detect with recent methods 1000 HBV DNA copies per mL of serum. Previous methods (branched DNA testing) could detect 1 000 000 HBV DNA copies per mL. Different assays are not standardized and so far provide different results on the same specimen. In the more recent studies the median of viral load ranged from 2 to 4 million copies per mL.

Testing sensitive HBV DNA is particularly useful when: transaminases are normal, several causes of liver disease are possible (ie, alcohol consumption), and in immunosuppressed patients (ie, after transplantation, in HIV-coinfected patients).

Precore/core variability

Two different transcripts, the precore and the core, are translated into the hepatitis B e (HBe) and core (HBc) proteins, respectively, also referred as HBeAg and HBcAg.

Genotype and serotype

There are seven genotypes of hepatitis B (from A to G) and four standard HBsAg subtypes (adr, adw, ayw and ayr). The clinical significance of HBV genotypes and serotypes is largely unknown.

References

1   Blumberg BS, Alter HJ, Visnik S. A "new" antigen in leukemia sera. *JAMA* 1965; **191**: 541–46.

2   Szmuness W, Stevens CE, Hadler SC. Hepatitis B: evolving epidemiology and implications for control. *Semin Liver Dis* 1991; **11**: 84–92.

3   Maddrey WC. Hepatitis B: an important public health issue. *Clin Lab* 2001; **47**: 51–55.

4   Carman WF, Jacyna MR, Hadziyannis S, et al. Mutation preventing formation of hepatitis e antigen in patients with chronic hepatitis B infection. *Lancet* 1989; **ii**: 588–91.

5   Bonino F, Brunetto MR, Rizetto M, et al. Hepatitis B virus unable to secrete e antigen. *Gastroenterology* 1991; **100**: 1138–41.

6   Zarski JP, Marcellin P, Cohard M, et al. Comparison of anti-HBe-positive and HBe-antigen-positive chronic hepatitis B in France: French Multicentre Group. *J Hepatol* 1994; **20**: 636–40.

7   Sanchez-Tapias JM. Natural history of chronic hepatitis B. In: Buti M, Esteban R, Guardia J, eds. Viral hepatitis. Barcelona: Accion Medica, 2000; 21–31.

8   Lok ASF. Hepatitis B infection: pathogenesis and management. *J Hepatol* 2000; **32**: 89–97.

9   Takeda K, Akahane Y, Suzuki H, et al. Defects in the precore region of the HBV genome in patients with chronic hepatitis B after sustained seroconversion from HBeAg to anti-HBe induced

spontaneously or with interferon therapy. *Hepatology* 1990; **12**: 1284–89.

10 Brunetto MR, Giarin MM, Oliveri F, et al. Wild type and e antigen-minus hepatitis B viruses and course of chronic hepatitis. *Proc Natl Acad Sci USA* 1991; **88**: 4186–90.

11 Akarca US, Greene S, Lok ASF. Detection of precore hepatitis B virus mutants in asymptomatic HBsAg-positive family members. *Hepatology* 1994; **19**: 1366–70.

12 Villeneuve JP, Desrochers M, Infante-Rivard C, et al. A long-term follow-up study of asymptomatic hepatitis B surface antigen-positive carriers in Montreal. *Gastroenterology* 1994; **106**: 1000–05.

13 de Franchis R, Meucci G, Vecchi M, et al. The natural history of asymptomatic hepatitis B surface antigen carriers. *Ann Intern Med* 1993; **118**: 191–94.

14 Sakuma K, Takahara T, Okuda K, et al. Prognosis of hepatitis B virus surface antigen carriers in relation to routine liver function tests: a prospective study. *Gastroenterology* 1982; **83**: 114–17.

15 Tsubota A, Kumada H, Takaki K, et al. Deletions in the hepatitis B virus core gene may influence the clinical outcome in hepatitis B e antigen-positive asymptomatic healthy carriers. *J Med Virol* 1998; **56**: 287–93.

16 McMahon BJ, Alberts SR, Wainwright RB, et al. Hepatitis B-related sequelae: prospective study in 1400 hepatitis B surface antigen-positive Alaska native carriers. *Arch Intern Med* 1990; **150**: 1051–54.

17 Tainturier-Sayegh MH, Thibault V, Ratziu V, et al. Is it possible to reduce liver biopsy indication in HBsAG positive patients with undetectable HBV-DNA? *Hepatology* 2000; **32**: 452A.

18 Poynard T, Mathurin P, Lai CL, et al. Natural history of fibrosis progression in chronic liver diseases. *Hepatology* 2000; **32**: 109A.

19 Huo TI, Wu JC, Lee PC, et al. Sero-clearance of hepatitis B surface antigen in chronic carriers does not necessarily imply a good prognosis. *Hepatology* 1998; **28**: 231–36.

20 Lai ME, Solinas A, Mazzoleni AP, et al. The role of pre-core hepatitis B virus mutants on the long-term outcome of chronic hepatitis B virus hepatitis: a longitudinal study. *J Hepatol* 1994; **20**: 773–81.

21 Lai CL, Chien RN, Leung N, et al. Lamivudine therapy for chronic hepatitis B: a 12 month double-blind, placebo-controlled multicentre study. *N Engl J Med* 1998; **339**: 61–68.

22 Bortolotti F, Jara P, Crivellaro C, et al. Outcome of chronic hepatitis B in Caucasian children during a 20-year observation period. *J Hepatol* 1998; **29**: 184–88.

23 Okuda K. Early recognition of hepatocellular carcinoma. *Hepatology* 1986; **6**: 729–38.

24 Bosch X. Global epidemiology of hepatocellular carcinoma. In: K Okuda, E Tabor, eds. Liver cancer. New York: Churchill Livingstone, 1997: 13–28.

25 Beasley RP, Hwang LY, Lin CC, et al. Hepatocellular carcinoma and hepatitis B virus: a prospective study of 22 707 men in Taiwan. *Lancet* 1981; **ii**: 1129–33.

26 Brechot C, Hadchouel M, Scotto J, et al. State of hepatitis B virus DNA, in hepatocytes of patients with HBsAg positive and HBsAg negative liver diseases. *Proc Natl Acad Sci USA* 1981; **78**: 3906–10.

27 Poper H, Shih JW, Gerin JL, et al. Woodchuck hepatitis and hepatocellular carcinoma: correlation of histological and virological observations. *Hepatology* 1981; **1**: 91–98.

28 El-Serag HB, Mason A. Rising incidence of hepatocellular carcinoma in the United States. *N Engl J Med* 1999; **34**: 745–50.

29 Chang MH, Chen CJ, Lai MS, et al. Universal hepatitis B vaccination in Taiwan and the incidence of hepatocellular carcinoma in children. *N Engl J Med* 1997; **336**: 1855–59.

30 Chen PJ, Chen DS. Hepatitis B virus infection and hepatocellular carcinoma: molecular genetics and clinical perspectives. *Semin Liver Dis* 1999; **19**: 253–62.

31 Cacciola I, Pollicino T, Squadrito G, et al. Occult hepatitis B virus infection in patients with chronic hepatitis C liver disease. *N Engl J Med* 1999; **341**: 22–26.

32 Yamamoto K, Horikita M, Tsuda F, et al. Naturally occurring escape mutants of hepatitis B virus with various mutations in the S gene in carriers seropositive for antibody to hepatitis B surface antigen. *J Virol* 1994; **68**: 2671–76.

33 Rehermann B, Ferrari C, Pasquinelli C, Chisari FV. The hepatitis B virus persists for decades after patients' recovery from acute viral hepatitis despite active maintenance of a cytotoxic T-lymphocyte response. *Nat Med* 1996; **2**: 1104–08.

34 Trepo C, Thivolet J. Antigène Australia antigen, virus de l'hepatite et periarterite noueuse. *Presse Med* 1970; **78**: 1575.

35 Willson RA. Extrahepatic manifestations of chronic viral hepatitis. In: Wilson RA, ed. *Viral Hepatitis, Diagnostic, Treatment, Prevention.* New York: Marcel Dekker, 1997: 331–69.

36 Pyrsopoulos NT, Reddy KR. Extrahepatic manifestations of chronic viral hepatitis. *Curr Gastroenterol Rep* 2001; **3**: 71–78.

37 Lhote F, Cohen P, Guillevin L. Polyarteritis nodosa, microscopic polyangiitis and Churg-Strauss syndrome. *Lupus* 1998; **7**: 238–58.

38 Guillevin L, Lhote F, Cohen P, et al. Polyarteritis nodosa related to hepatitis B virus: a prospective study with long-term observation of 41 patients. *Medicine (Baltimore)* 1995; **74**: 238–53.

39 Zurn A, Schmied E, Saurat JH. Cutaneous manifestations of infection due to hepatitis B virus. *Schweiz Rundsch Med Prax* 1990; **79**: 1254–57.

40 Johnson RJ, Gouser WG. Hepatitis B infection and renal disease: clinical, immunopathogenic and therapeutic considerations. *Kidney Int* 1990; **37**: 663–76.

41 Lunel F, Musset L, Cacoub P, et al. Cryoglobulinemia in chronic liver diseases: role of hepatitis C virus and liver damage. *Gastroenterology* 1994; **106**: 1291–300.

42 Foster GR, Goldin RD, Thomas HC. Chronic hepatitis C virus infection causes a significant reduction in quality of life in the absence of cirrhosis. *Hepatology* 1998; **27**: 209–12.

43 Owens DK, Cardinalli AB, Nease RF. Physicians' assessments of the utility of health states associated with human immunodeficiency virus (HIV) and hepatitis B virus (HBV) infection. *Qual Life Res* 1997; **6**: 77–86.

44 Hoofnagle JH, di Bisceglie AM. The treatment of chronic viral hepatitis. *N Engl J Med* 1997; **336**: 347–56.

45 Wong DK, Cheung AM, O'Rourke K, et al. Effect of alpha-interferon treatment in patients with hepatitis B e antigen-positive chronic hepatitis B: a meta-analysis. *Ann Intern Med* 1993; **119**: 312–23.

46 Brook MG, Petrovic L, McDonald JA, et al. Histological improvement after anti-viral treatment for chronic hepatitis B virus infection. *J Hepatol* 1989; **8**: 218–25.

47 Niederau C, Heintges T, Lange S, et al. Long-term follow-up of HBeAg-positive patients treated with interferon alfa for chronic hepatitis B. *N Engl J Med* 1996; **334**: 1422–27.

48 Lin SM, Sheen IS, Chien RN, et al. Long-term beneficial effect of interferon therapy in patients with chronic hepatitis B virus infection. *Hepatology* 1999; **29**: 971–75.

49 Perrillo R, Tamburro C, Regenstein F, et al. Low-dose, titratable interferon alpha in decompensated liver disease caused by chronic infection with hepatitis B virus. *Gastroenterology* 1995; **109**: 908–16.

50 Benhamou Y, Dohin E, Lunel-Fabiani F, et al. Efficacy of lamivudine on replication of hepatitis B virus in HIV-infected patients. *Lancet* 1995; **345**: 396–97.

51 Benhamou Y, Katlama C, Lunel F, et al. The effects of lamivudine on replication of hepatitis B virus in HIV-infected men. *Ann Intern Med* 1996; **125**: 705–12.

52 Benhamou Y, Bochet M, Thibault V, et al. Long term incidence of hepatitis B virus resistance to lamivudine in HIV-infected patients. *Hepatology* 1999; **30**: 1302–06.

53 Dienstag JL, Perrillo RP, Schiff ER, et al. A preliminary trial of lamivudine for chronic hepatitis B infection. *N Engl J Med* 1995; **333**: 1657–61.

54 Lai CL, Chien RN, Leung NWY, et al. A one year trial of lamivudine for chronic hepatitis B. *N Engl J Med* 1998; **339**: 61–68.

55 Dienstag JL, Schiff ER, Wright T, et al. Lamivudine as initial treatment for chronic hepatitis B in the United States. *N Engl J Med* 1999; **341**: 1256–63.

56 Tassopoulos NC, Volpes R, Pastore G, et al. Efficacy of lamivudine in patients with hepatitis B e antigen-negative/hepatitis B virus DNA-positive (precore mutant) chronic hepatitis B. *Hepatology* 1999; **29**: 889–96.

57 Perillo R. Multicenter study of lamivudine therapy for hepatitis B after liver transplantation: lamivudine transplant group. *Hepatology* 1999; **29**: 1581–86.

58 Yao FY, Bass NM. Lamivudine treatment in patients with severely decompensated cirrhosis due to replicating hepatitis B infection. *J Hepatol* 2000; **33**: 301–07.

59 Liaw YF, Lai CL, Leung NWY, et al. Effects of extended lamivudine therapy in Asian patients with chronic hepatitis B. *Gastroenterology* 2000; **119**: 172–80.

60 Chayama K, Suzuki Y, Kobayashi M, et al. Emergence and takeover of YMDD motif mutant hepatitis B virus during long-term lamivudine therapy and re-takeover by wild type after cessation of therapy. *Hepatology* 1998; **27**: 1711–16.

61 Allen MI, Deslauriers M, Andrews CW, et al. Identification and characterization of mutations in hepatitis B virus resistant to lamivudine: Lamivudine Clinical Investigation Group. *Hepatology* 1998; **27**: 1670–77.

62 Zollner B, Petersen J, Schroter M, et al. 20-fold increase in risk of lamivudine resistance in hepatitis B virus subtype adw. *Lancet* 2001; **357**: 934–35.

63 Schalm SW, Heathcote J, Cianciara J, et al. Lamivudine and alpha interferon combination treatment of patients with chronic hepatitis B infection: a randomised trial. *Gut* 2000; **46**: 562–68.

64 Xiong K, Flores C, Yang H, et al. Mutations in hepatitis B DNA polymerase associated with resistance to lamivudine do not confer resistance to adefovir *in vitro*. *Hepatology* 1998; **28**: 1669–73.

65 Gilson RJ, Chopra KB, Newell AM, et al. A placebo-controlled phase I/II study of adefovir dipivoxil in patients with chronic hepatitis B virus infection. *J Viral Hepatitis* 1999; **6**: 387–95.

66 Peters MG, Singer G, Howard T, et al. Fulminant hepatic failure resulting from lamivudine-resistant hepatitis B virus in a renal transplant recipient: durable response after orthotopic liver transplantation on adefovir dipivoxil and hepatitis B immune globulin. *Transplantation* 1999; **68**: 1912–14.

67 Perrillo R, Schiff E, Yoshida E, et al. Adefovir dipivoxil for the treatment of lamivudine-resistant hepatitis B mutants. *Hepatology* 2000; **32**: 129–34.

68 Benhamou Y, Bochet M, Thibault V, et al. An open label pilot study of the safety and efficacy of adefovir dipivoxil in HIV/HBV co-infected patients with lamivudine resistant HBV. *Lancet* (in press).

69 Ono SK, Kato N, Shiratori Y, et al. The polymerase L528M mutation cooperates with nucleotide binding-site mutations, increasing hepatitis B virus replication and drug resistance. *J Clin Invest* 2001; **107**: 449–55.

70 Rizzetto M, Volpes R, Smedile A. Response of pre-core mutant chronic hepatitis B infection to lamivudine. *J Med Virol* 2000; **61**: 398–400.

71 Shouval D, Samuel D. Hepatitis B immune globulin to prevent hepatitis B virus graft reinfection following liver transplantation: a concise review. *Hepatology* 2000; **32**: 1189–95.

72 Colquhoun SD, Belle SH, Samuel D, et al. Transplantation in the hepatitis B patient and current therapies to prevent recurrence. *Semin Liver Dis* 2000; **20**(suppl 1): 7–12.

73 Perrillo RP, Wright T, Rakela J, et al. A multicenter United States–Canadian trial to assess lamivudine monotherapy before and after liver transplantation for chronic hepatitis B. *Hepatology* 2001; **33**: 424–32.

74 Han SH, Ofman J, Holt C, et al. An efficacy and cost-effectiveness analysis of combination hepatitis B immune globulin and lamivudine to prevent recurrent hepatitis B after orthotopic liver transplantation compared with hepatitis B immune globulin monotherapy. *Liver Transpl* 2000; **6**: 741–48.

75 Crowley SJ, Tognarini D, Desmond PV, Lees M. Cost-effectiveness analysis of lamivudine for the treatment of chronic hepatitis B. *Pharmacoeconomics* 2000; **17**: 409–27.

Hepatitis C

Natural history of hepatitis C: Epidemiology

It took many years before communities realized the importance of the hepatitis C epidemic (Figure 17.1).

Chronic hepatitis C virus (HCV) infection is estimated to affect 170 million individuals worldwide (Figure 17.2).[1] These individuals are at risk of developing hepatological and non-hepatological manifestations.

Hepatitis C can cause cirrhosis, digestive haemorrhage, liver failure, and liver cancer. Hepatitis C is the major reason for liver transplants together with alcoholic cirrhosis in Europe and in the United States. Cumulative evidence

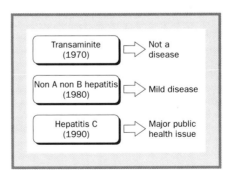

Figure 17.1
Perception of HCV epidemic.

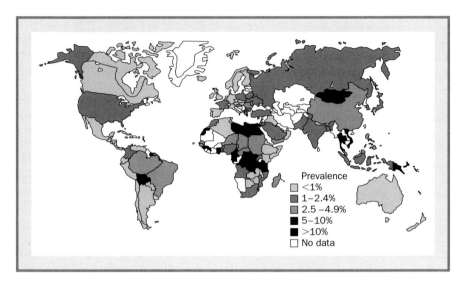

Figure 17.2
World prevalence of HCV in 1997.

strongly suggests that the increase of mortality due to hepatocellular carcinoma in most western countries is because of hepatitis C infection (Figures 17.3 and 17.4).[2–5]

Transmission of HCV is mainly related to contact with blood and blood products (Table 17.1). Blood transfusions and the use of shared, non-sterilized needles and syringes have been the main causes of the spread of HCV. With routine blood screening for HCV antibody (since 1991 in most countries) transfusion-related hepatitis C has virtually disappeared. At present, intravenous drug use is the most common risk factor. However, many other patients acquire HCV without any known exposure to blood or to drug injection. A recent survey suggests that patients with high-risk sexual behaviour are at higher risk, perhaps associated with herpes simplex 2 infection.[6]

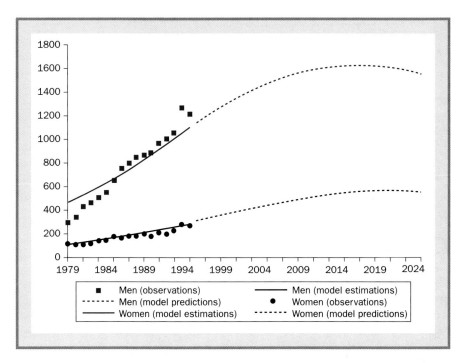

Figure 17.3
Increase in mortality related to primary liver cancer because of hepatitis C in France. Adapted with permission.[4]

Table 17.1 Risk groups for HCV infection.

Major high-risk groups	*Blood transfusion before 1991* *Frequent exposure to blood products: haemophilia, transplants, haemodialysis, chronic renal failure, gammaglobulins, cancer chemotherapy.* *Intravenous drug users, even briefly and many years ago.* *Health-care workers with needle-stick accidents.* *Infants born to HCV-infected mothers particularly those coinfected by HIV.*
Moderate-risk groups	*High-risk sexual behaviour, multiple partners, history of herpes simplex 2 infection.* *Cocaine use, with sharing of intranasal administration equipment.*

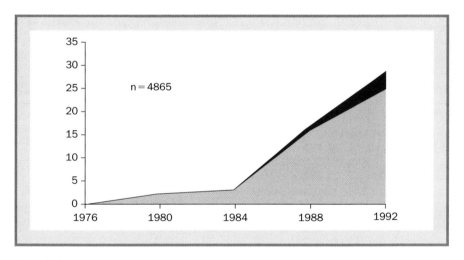

Figure 17.4
Increase in mortality related to primary liver cancer and liver disease in UK haemophilia population. Adapted with permission.[4]

Natural history of hepatitis C: Hepatic manifestations

18

The major hepatological consequence of HCV infection is the progression to cirrhosis and its potential complications: haemorrhage, hepatic insufficiency, and primary liver cancer.

Current understanding of HCV infection has been advanced by the concept of liver fibrosis progression (Figure 18.1).[7,8] Fibrosis is the deleterious but variable consequence of chronic inflammation; it is characterized by the deposition of extracellular matrix component leading to the distortion of the hepatic architecture with impairment of liver microcirculation and liver cell functions. HCV is usually only lethal when it leads to cirrhosis, the last stage of liver fibrosis. Therefore, an estimate of fibrosis progression represents an important surrogate endpoint for assessment of the vulnerability of an individual patient and for assessment of the impact of treatment on natural history.

Fibrosis stages and necroinflammatory activity grades

Activity and fibrosis are two major histological features of chronic hepatitis C that are included in different proposed classifications.[9–12] One of the few validated scoring systems is

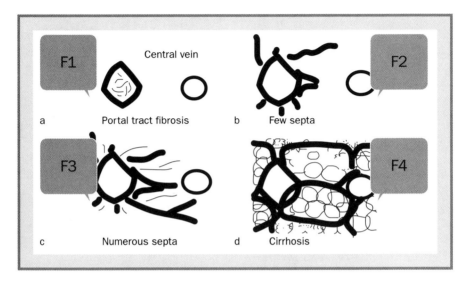

Figure 18.1
The METAVIR fibrosis staging system. F0 is normal liver (no fibrosis); a) F1 = portal tract fibrosis; b) F2 = few septa; c) F3 = numerous septa; d) F4 = cirrhosis.

called the METAVIR scoring system.[11,12] This system assesses histological lesions in chronic hepatitis C by the use of two separate scores, one for necroinflammatory grade (A for activity) and another for the stage of fibrosis (F). These scores were defined as follows. Stages of fibrosis (F) (Figure 18.2):

F0 = no fibrosis,

F1 = portal fibrosis without septa,

F2 = portal fibrosis with rare septa,

F3 = numerous septa without cirrhosis,

F4 = cirrhosis.

Grade for activity (A): A0 = no histological activity, A1 = minimal activity, A2 = moderate activity, A3 = severe activity. The degree of activity was assessed by integration of the severity of the intensity of both piecemeal (periportal) necrosis and lobular necrosis as described in a simple algorithm.[12] The intra-observer and inter-observer variations of this METAVIR scoring system are lower than those of the widely used Knodell scoring system.[9,10] For METAVIR fibrosis stages there is an almost perfect concordance ($\kappa = 0.80$) among pathologists. The Knodell scoring system has a non-linear scale. There is no stage 2 for fibrosis (range predictive of fibrosis progression independently of fibrosis stage.[14] Fibrosis stage and inflammatory grade are correlated but, for one third of patients, there is discordance. The clinician should not take a "significant activity" as a surrogate marker of "a severe disease". The clinical hallmarks of major necrosis and inflammation (ie, severe acute hepatitis and fulminant hepatitis) are very rare in comparison to hepatitis B. Even in immunologically compromised patients there are very few acute flare-ups in patients with chronic hepatitis C.

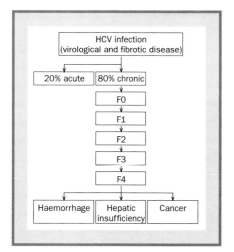

Figure 18.2
The model of fibrosis progression from infection to complications. Estimated key numbers of HCV natural history from literature and our database. Median time from infection (F0) to cirrhosis (F4) is 30 years. Mortality at 10 years for cirrhosis is 50%. Transition probability per year from non-complicated cirrhosis to each of the complications is around 3%.

The dynamic view of fibrosis progression

Fibrosis stage summarizes the vulnerability of a patient and is predictive of the progression to cirrhosis (Figure 18.2).[6] There is a strong correlation for fibrosis stages, almost linear, with age at biopsy and duration of infection. This correlation was not observed between activity grades.

Because of the informative value of fibrosis stage there is a reason for the clinician to assess the speed of the fibrosis progression. The distribution of fibrosis progression rates suggests the presence of at least three populations: one population of "rapid fibrosers", a population of "intermediate fibrosers", and one population of "slow fibrosers" (Figure 18.3). Therefore the expressions of a mean (or median) fibrosis progression rate per year (stage at the first

0–4) and the activity grade ranges from 0 to 18 with the sum of periportal necrosis, intralobular and portal inflammation grades. The modified Histological Activity Index is more detailed with four different features and continuous grades and the modified fibrosis staging includes six stages.

Activity grade, which represents the necrosis feature, is not a good predictor of fibrosis progression.[7] In fact fibrosis alone is the best marker of ongoing fibrogenesis.[13] So far there is no study showing clearly that activity grades are

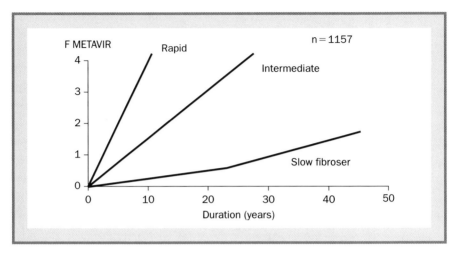

Figure 18.3
Progression of liver fibrosis in patients with chronic hepatitis C. By use of median fibrosis progression rate, in untreated patients, median expected time to cirrhosis is 30 years (intermediate fibroser). 33% of patients have expected median time to cirrhosis of less than 20 years (rapid fibroser). 31% will progress to cirrhosis in more than 50 years, if ever (slow fibroser). Adapted with permission.[7]

biopsy/duration of infection) and of a mean expected time to cirrhosis does not signify that the progression to cirrhosis is universal and inevitable. By use of the median fibrosis progression rate, in untreated patients, the median expected time to cirrhosis is 30 years; 33% of patients have an expected median time to cirrhosis of less than 20 years and 31% will progress to cirrhosis in more than 50 years, if ever (Figure 18.3).

Limitations of any estimate of fibrosis include: the difficulty in obtaining paired liver biopsies; the necessity for large numbers of patients to achieve statistical power; and the sample variability in fibrosis distribution. Because the time elapsed between biopsies is short (usually between 12 to 24 months), the number of events (transition from one stage to another) is rare. Therefore the comparisons between fibrosis progression rates require a large sample size to observe significant differences. The slope of progression is difficult to assess because there is no large database with several biopsies. Therefore the real slope is currently unknown and, even if there is a linear relationship between stages and age at biopsy or duration of infection, other models are possible.[15] We recently

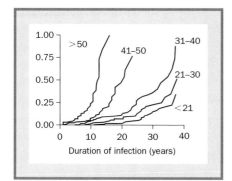

Figure 18.4
Probability of fibrosis progression to cirrhosis (F4) according to age at infection. Modelling in 2313 patients with known duration of infection. Adapted with permission.[16]

confirmed on a larger database that fibrosis progression was mainly dependent on the age and the duration of infection with four different periods with very slow, slow, intermediate, and rapid slopes (Figure 18.4).[16]

Furthermore liver biopsy has its own limits in assessing liver fibrosis. Although it is the gold standard to score fibrosis, its value is limited by sample variability. At least a 10 mm length biopsy is mandatory to accurately assess fibrosis.

Factors associated with fibrosis progression

Factors associated and not associated with fibrosis are summarized in Table 18.1. Several factors have been clearly shown to be associated with fibrosis progression rate:[4,7,16–19] duration of infection, age, male sex, consumption of alcohol, HIV coinfection, and low CD4 count. The progression from infection to cirrhosis depends strongly on sex, age, and alcohol consumption (Table 18.2).[4,7]

Table 18.1 Factors associated or not with fibrosis progression.

Associated in univariate and multivariate analysis	Not sure	Not associated
Age at infection	Necrosis	Last serum viral load
Duration of infection	Inflammation	Genotype
Age at biopsy	Haemochromatosis heterozygote	Mode of infection
Consumption of alcohol >50 g per day	Cigarette consumption	DR antigens
HIV coinfection	Steatosis	Liver viral load
CD4 count <200 mL	Body mass index	HCV-HVR1 complexity
Female sex	Moderate alcohol consumption	
Fibrosis stage	Diabetes	

Table 18.2 Multivariate analysis of risk factors by proportional-hazards regression model for each fibrosis stage 20 years after HCV infection in 2313 patients. Adapted with permission.[16]

Risk factor	Stage F1		Stage F2		Stage F3		Stage F4	
	Relative hazard	p	Relative hazard	p	Relative hazard	p	Relative hazard	p
Infection after 30 years	4.4	<0.001	4.8	<0.001	11.5	<0.001	27.1	<0.001
Infection 21–30 years	2.3	<0.001	1.8	<0.001	2.5	<0.001	5.3	<0.001
Alcohol >50 g	1.3	0.20	3.0	<0.001	2.3	0.008	4.5	0.001
Male	1.0	0.76	1.3	0.03	1.9	<0.001	2.0	0.003
Intravenous drug user	1.6	<0.001	1.2	0.22	1.4	0.11	1.2	0.55
Activity A2, A3	0.8	0.009	1.2	0.21	2.0	<0.001	1.4	0.16

Age

The role of ageing in fibrosis progression could be related to higher vulnerability to environmental factors, especially oxidative stress, to reduction in blood flow, in mitochondria capacity, or in immune capacities.[20]

The effect of age on fibrosis progression is so important that modelling the hepatitis C epidemic without taking into account age is not possible. The estimated probability of progression per year for men aged between 61 and 70 years was 300 times greater than that for men aged between 21 and 40 years (Figure 18.4).[4,16]

Female sex

Female sex is associated with ten times less rapid progression to cirrhosis than in males, whatever the age.[19] Oestrogen modulates fibrogenesis in experimental injury. Oestrogen blocks proliferation and fibrogenesis by stellate cells in primary culture. Oestrogen could be modifying the expression of transforming growth factor and other soluble mediators.

Alcohol

The role of alcohol consumption has been established for daily doses greater than 40 or 50 g per day.[7,16,17] For lower doses there are discordant results with even preliminary studies suggesting a protective effect of very small doses. Alcohol consumption is difficult to quantify and conclusions must be prudent. However, it seems from these studies that the influence of alcohol is independent of other factors, weaker compared with age, and is exerted only at toxic levels of intake.

HIV coinfection

Several studies have shown that patients coinfected with HCV and HIV have a faster fibrosis progression rate than controls even after taking into account age, sex, and alcohol consumption (Figure 18.5a).[18,21] An HIV-infected patient with less than 200 CD4 cells/μL and drinking more than 50 g of alcohol daily has a median expected time to cirrhosis of 16 years versus 36 years for an HIV-infected patient with more than 200 CD4 cells/μL, drinking 50 g or less of alcohol daily (Figure 18.5b).

Viral factors

Viral factors such as genotype, viral load at the time of the biopsy, and quasi species are not associated with fibrosis.[7,22,23] There are very few studies for the following factors and more studies with high sample size are needed: fluctuations of HCV RNA, intrahepatic cytokines profiles, HLA class genotype, C282Y heterozygote hemochromatosis gene mutation, and cigarette consumption.

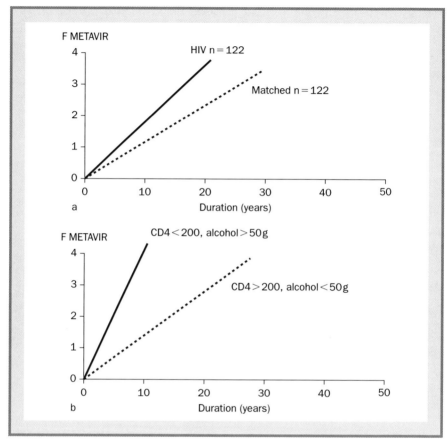

Figure 18.5
Progression of liver fibrosis among patients coinfected by HCV and HIV. a) There is significant increase of fibrosis progression rate among HIV in comparison with matched controls infected by HCV alone. Adapted with permission.[18] b) There is very significant increase of fibrosis progression rate among patients with CD4 <200 per mL and drinking more than 50 g of alcohol per day. Adapted with permission.[18]

Risk of fibrosis in patients with normal transaminases

Patients with repeated normal serum transaminase activity have a lower fibrosis progression rate than matched control patients with elevated transaminases (Figure 18.6).[24] However, there is still 15% of these patients with moderate or high fibrosis progression rates. Therefore, we recommend performing liver biopsy in these PCR-positive patients. If the patient has septal fibrosis or portal fibrosis with a high fibrosis rate a treatment should be considered.

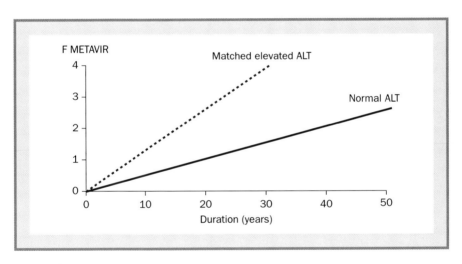

Figure 18.6
Progression of liver fibrosis in patients HCV PCR positive with repeated normal transaminases ALT. There was a significant reduction of fibrosis progression rate in comparison with matched controls with abnormal transaminases ALT. Adapted with permission.[24]

Natural history of hepatitis C: Extra-hepatic manifestations

19

Numerous extrahepatic manifestations have been reported with HCV infection including fatigue, mixed cryoglobulinaemia, porphyria cutanea tarda, membranous glomerulonephritis, sicca syndrome, thyroiditis, and high prevalence of autoantibodies.[25] We analysed a cross-sectional study including 1614 patients;[26] overall prevalence of the extrahepatic manifestations is shown in Table 19.1. By multivariate analysis, three main risk factors were associated with the presence of clinical or biological extrahepatic manifestations: advanced age, female sex, and extensive liver fibrosis. There was no association with histological activity grade.

Clinical manifestations

The extrahepatic clinical manifestations are particularly frequent, 74% of patients (95% CI 72–77) presenting at least one, with a preponderance of rheumatic (ie, arthralgia, myalgia, paresthesia) and cutaneomucous (pruritus, sicca syndrome, Raynaud's phenomenon) symptoms. Six manifestations had a prevalence above 10% including, in decreasing order, fatigue, arthralgia, paresthesia, myalgia,

Table 19.1 Prevalence of clinical and biological extrahepatic manifestations in HCV positive patients (decreasing order). Adapted with permission.[25]

	%	95% CI
Clinical extrahepatic manifestation*		
Fatigue	53	51–56
Arthralgia	23	21–26
Paresthesia	17	15–19
Myalgia	15	14–17
Pruritus	15	13–17
Sicca syndrome	11	10–13
Arterial hypertension	10	8–11
Diabetes	7	5–8
Raynaud's phenomenon	3.5	2.6–4.5
Abnormal thyroid function	3.4	2.0–4.0
Psoriasis	3	2–4
At least one clinical manifestation	74	72–77
Biological extrahepatic manifestation†		
Cryoglobulin (1083)	40	37–43
Anti-nuclear Ab (874)	10	8–12
Low thyroxin (661)	10	8–13
Antismooth muscle Ab (873)	7	5–9
Antimicrosomal thyroid Ab (451)	5	3–8
Elevated creatininaemia (1614)	3	2–4

Ab = antibodies.
The following extrahepatic manifestations were present in less than 2% of patients: purpura 1.5%, vasculitis 1%, lichen planus 1%, porphyria cutanea tarda 0.2%, antithyroglobulin Ab 2%, antiliver-kidney microsomal Ab 2%, antimitochondrial Ab 1%, elevated thyroid stimulating hormone 1%, low thyroid-stimulating hormone 1%, elevated thyroxin 1%.
* Tested in 1614 patients; † total tested given in parentheses.

pruritus, and sicca syndrome. This may reflect non-specific prevalence of these symptoms, because there is no control population matched for age and sex. Systemic lupus erythematosus, Sjögren's syndrome, rheumatoid arthritis, or dermatomyositis are uncommon in HCV positive patients, suggesting a fortuitous association. Systemic vasculitis, which is the severe symptomatic manifestation of cryoglobulinaemia, although rare (1%), is the most frequent systemic inflammatory disease observed.

Because of lymphotropism of HCV, a possible role of this viral agent has been suggested in the development of haemolymphopathies, in particular B-cell non-Hodgkin's lymphoma in patients with HCV-mixed cryoglobulinaemia.[27] Only one out of 1614 HCV patients in our cohort has developed a non-Hodgkin's lymphoma to date.[26]

Biological manifestations

Four biological abnormalities have a prevalence above 5%: cryoglobulin, antinuclear antibodies, antismooth muscle antibodies, and low thyroxin level. At least one biological abnormality is present in 50% of patients.[25,26]

Mixed cryoglobulins is the predominant extrahepatic biological manifestation, identified in 40% (95% CI 37–43) of the 1083 patients we tested. All cryoglobulin-positive patients had mixed type-II cryoglobulins (65%) or type III (35%). Five independent factors were significantly associated with the presence of a cryoglobulin: female sex, alcohol consumption above 50 g daily, HCV genotype 2 or 3, and extensive liver fibrosis. Cryoglobulin positive-patients present more arthralgia, arterial hypertension, purpura, and systemic vasculitis. However, given the high frequency of positive cryoglobulin in HCV patients, severely symptomatic mixed cryoglobulinaemia with

vasculitis is rare, noted in 2–3% of cryoglobulin-positive patients.

Most systematic searches for biological extrahepatic manifestation in HCV-infected patients revealed high prevalences of antinuclear (20–40%), antismooth muscle cell (20%), antithyroid (8–12%) and anticardiolipin (20%) antibodies. No association was observed between biological and clinical symptoms and autoantibodies positivity.

Numerous thyroid abnormalities have been observed among patients chronically infected by HCV, suggesting that HCV by itself or via an indirect immunological pathway may induce thyroid dysfunction.[28] In our experience, clinically relevant thyroid abnormalities at the first visit—that is before any interferon or other anti-HCV treatment—are rare. Low thyroxin levels are found in 10% of patients but elevated thyroid stimulating hormone levels are noted in only 1%. Prevalences of anti-thyroid antibodies are in accordance with the age and sex ratio of the population studied.

Health-related quality of life

One way to assess the clinical impact of hepatic and extra-hepatic manifestation among patients infected by HCV is to assess the health-related quality of life. Several studies have shown that even patients without cirrhosis have an impaired quality of life (Figure 19.1).[29–32] The quality of life is

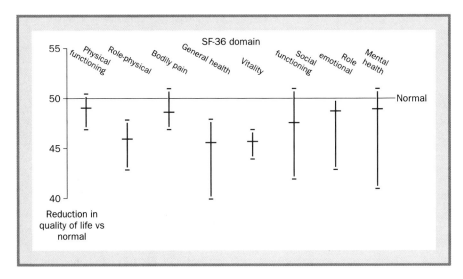

Figure 19.1
Quality of life impairment among patients infected with hepatitis C.

impaired by the diagnosis itself but also by the virus in comparison with controls.

Management protocols

In the past 10 years much progress has been made in the management of chronic hepatitis C, both in terms of viral endpoints and histological endpoints.

Worldwide approvals are not homogeneous across countries. Since the first approval in 1990 (standard interferon regimen monotherapy with three injections three times a week [TIW]) to the last approval in 2001

(combination of ribavirin and pegylated interferon) several main regimen have been assessed in large trials: standard interferon-alfa (alfa 2a or 2b, 3 MU TIW) for 24 weeks and then 48 weeks,[33,34] combination of standard interferon (3 MU TIW) and ribavirin (1000 mg ribavirin if weight <75 kg, 1200 mg ⩾ 75 kg) for 24 weeks or 48 weeks,[35–37] PEG interferon for 48 weeks (alfa 2a 180 µg, or alfa 2b at 3 doses: 0.5 µg, 1.0 µg, or 1.5 µg per kg),[38–40] and 48 weeks of combination PEG interferon and ribavirin (different doses of PEG and ribavirin).[41] Combination therapy was always more

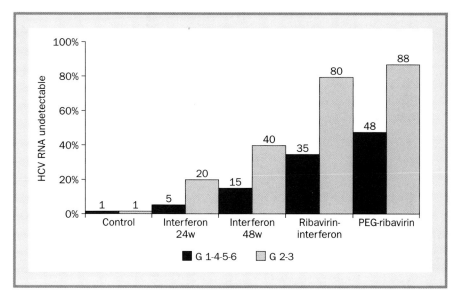

Figure 19.2
Progress in the treatment of chronic hepatitis C.

effective than interferon monotherapy, even PEG interferon monotherapy. The optimized combination regimen in the last European approval is the combination of 1.5 µg PEG interferon per kg and ribavirin adjusted on the weight as well: (800 mg if weight <65 kg, 1000 mg between 65 and 85 kg, and 1200 mg if weight >85 kg). A summary of the main progress is shown in Figure 19.2. Results were presented according to HCV genotype, the main factor associated with viral response.

Efficacy of ribavirin and standard interferon combination regimen

20

Efficacy of combination regimen on viral endpoints

When the two pivotal trials of ribavirin and interferon combination were combined,[35–37] the database included 1744 treatment-naïve patients. At the end of treatment, the percentage of patients with undetectable HCV RNA was significantly higher in the combination groups, 51% (260/505) in ribavirin-interferon week 48, 55% (278/505) in ribavirin-interferon week 24, 29% (147/503) in interferon week 48, and 29% in interferon week 24 (66/231), as shown in Figure 20.1a. At the end of the follow-up, the percentage of patients with sustained undetectable HCV RNA was also higher in the combination groups—41% (205/505), 33% (166/505), 16% (82/503), and 6% (13/231) respectively— with significant differences between all these groups (Figure 20.1b).

These results showed that there was a combination effect without duration effect on the end of treatment response and that there was a combination effect and a duration effect on the sustained response.

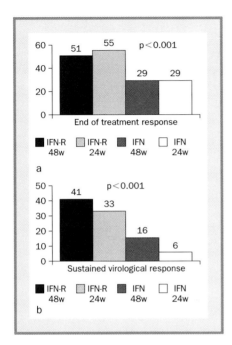

Figure 20.1
Efficacy of combination ribavirin-interferon at the end of the treatment (a) and at the end of 24 weeks follow-up (b).
Ribavirin 1.0–1.2 g + interferon 3 MU vs interferon 3 MU n = 1744 naïve patients

Efficacy of combination regimen on transaminase

There was a strong correlation between the impact of treatment on viral load and transaminases (Figures 20.2a and 20.2b). However, transaminase activity had a lower specificity for sustained response than viral load. 12% of patients with normal ALT at the end of follow-up were PCR positive.

Efficacy of combination regimen on histological endpoints

There was a significant improvement of activity grades (Figure 20.3a) and fibrosis progression rates (Figure 20.3b) when biopsies performed 24 weeks after the end of treatment were compared with baseline biopsies.[42] Improvement was greater in sustained responders.

Efficacy of combination regimen on extra-hepatic manifestations and on quality of life

Little is known concerning the efficacy of treatment on extra-hepatic manifestations. During the treatment and because of the adverse events there was an impairment of health-related quality of life in comparison with baseline value.[30,31] After the end of the treatment there was an improvement of health-related quality of life in sustained responders in comparison with baseline level.[30,31] In severe symptomatic cryoglobulinaemia there was a clinical improvement by treatment.

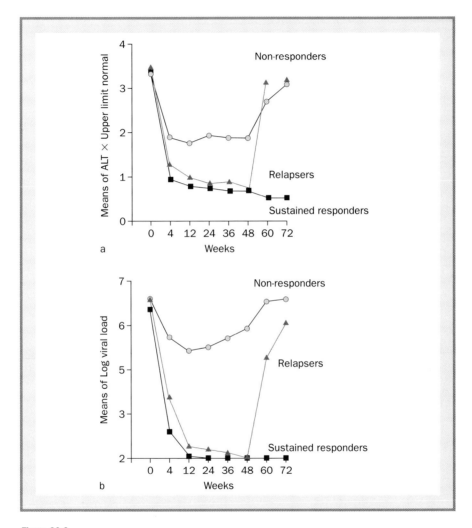

Figure 20.2
ALT a) and viral response b) to combination ribavirin-interferon in 536 patients treated 48 weeks.

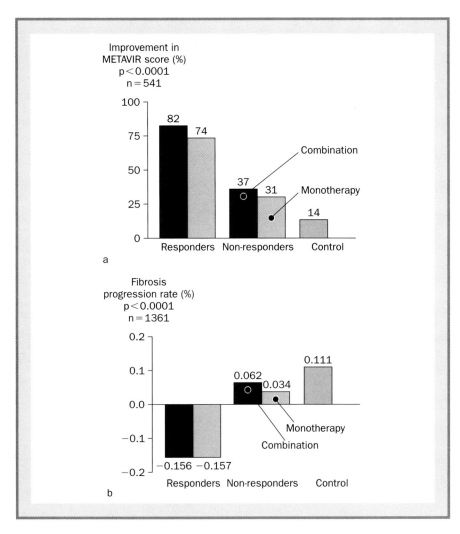

Figure 20.3
Improvement in histology after combination ribavirin-interferon. a) Activity grade. b) Fibrosis progression rate. Adapted with permission.[42]

Factors associated with treatment response and "à la carte" regimen

21

Careful analysis of pivotal trials has confirmed the independent prognostic values of five baseline characteristics.[37] HCV genotypes 2 and 3 were associated with better response to the combination than other genotypes. For viral load, the receiver operating characteristics (ROC) (Table 21.1) curves showed that there was no threshold that had either a positive or negative predictive value. Therefore, the simplest way to classify viral load as either high or low was to take the median, which was 3.5 million copies. For age, the threshold of 40 years seemed to be the most accurate. Because the multivariate analysis showed that these five factors could only explain 20% of the variability of the sustained response, we need to identify the other independent factors. These analyses have excluded the fact that the kinetics of viral load at 4 weeks and 12 weeks allow us to take a very early therapeutic decision. Furthermore, the antifibrotic effect of 24 weeks treatment in non-responders is a benefit for patients.[44]

Table 21.1 Sustained virological response to different regimens according to baseline characteristics.

Baseline characteristic	Ribavirin-interferon	
	48 weeks	**24 weeks**
Genotype		
2 or 3	65%	67%
1, 4, 5, or 6	30%	18%
Mean HCV RNA		
$\leq 3.5 \times 10^6$ copies/mL	44%	40%
$>3.5 \times 10^6$ copies/mL	38%	26%
Age		
≤ 40 years	48%	40%
>40 years	34%	26%
Fibrosis stage		
No or portal fibrosis	43%	36%
Septal fibrosis or more	36%	23%
Gender		
Female	46%	39%
Male	38%	30%
Combination of virological factors		
Genotype 2,3 $\leq 3.5 \times 10^6$	65%	71%
Genotype 2,3 $>3.5 \times 10^6$	65%	62%
Genotype 1,4,5,6 $\leq 3.5 \times 10^6$	33%	26%
Genotype 1,4,5,6 $>3.5 \times 10^6$	27%	10%
Combination of non-virological factors		
Woman ≤ 40 years, no or portal fibrosis	57%	56%
Men >40 years, septal fibrosis or more	34%	25%
Extremely favourable population		
Woman ≤ 40 years, no or portal fibrosis		
genotype 2,3 $\leq 3.5 \times 10^6$	79%	69%
Extremely unfavourable population		
Men >40 years, septal fibrosis or more,		
genotype 1,4,5,6 $>3.5 \times 10^6$	9%	8%

Is treatment by interferon alone sufficient among patients with many beneficial factors?

There is no place for interferon monotherapy at a dose of 3 million units three times a week for either 24 or 48 weeks even in a patient with many beneficial factors. Among patients with genotype 2 or 3 and low viral load, the sustained response rate was much greater with 24 weeks combination regimen (71%) than with 48 weeks of interferon monotherapy (40% p < 0.001). Interferon monotherapy should be recommended only if combination interferon alfa-2b plus ribavirin therapy is contraindicated.

Duration of combination regimen: 12, 24, or 48 weeks?

The first question is whether treatment can be stopped at 12 weeks in some subgroups because of a high probability of non-response. There was no consensus at an international conference.[43] From our data this approach cannot be recommended because in the 48-week regimen, among the patients who had a positive PCR at 12 weeks, we observed a sustained response in 10% of patients. Even 24 weeks regimen induces a sustained response in 4% of these patients.

Furthermore, the antifibrotic effect of 24 weeks treatment in non-responders is a benefit for patients.[44]

The choice of 24 weeks or 48 weeks for combination therapy has been clarified. The crucial time to make this decision is at 24 weeks based on the results of HCV PCR testing. In patients who are PCR negative at 24 weeks (59% of the patients in these studies), the goal is to reduce the relapse rate. There was an overall highly significant improvement with 48 weeks of treatment (74% sustained responders) versus 24 weeks (59% sustained responders). Since patients with many beneficial response factors benefit less from 48 weeks of treatment, consideration can be given to stopping at 24 weeks in these patients. A simple strategy could be to consider only the HCV genotype, and stop treatment at week 24 in genotype 2 and 3 responders, since the sustained response was 82% in patients treated 24 weeks versus 84% in patients treated 48 weeks. However, from our results it seems hazardous to recommend a strategy based only on virological characteristics. There were in fact five independent response factors, and to take into account only one factor among these five is an over-simplification that could lead to errors in different populations or subgroups.[37] For example, we have identified that patients with genotype 2 or 3 who are PCR negative at 24 weeks and who have extensive fibrosis will have a better sustained response with 48 weeks of treatment, 80%, compared with 65% in patients whose treatment is stopped at 24 weeks. For a population of older men with extensive fibrosis, the choice of 48 weeks duration in responders should not be based only on genotype and viral load. The recommendation of the international consensus conference to treat patients with genotype 2 or 3 for only 24 weeks, irrespective of the other factors, seems inappropriate.[43] Furthermore, from a clinical point of view there is the risk of oversimplifying a decision according to a specific threshold, ie, choice of 48 weeks treatment if the viral load is 3.75 million and 24 weeks if 3.25 million or 39 versus 41 years of age. This argues for taking the decision on both the number of independent factors and the tolerance to the combination.

Similarly, the recommendation of the international consensus conference[43] to treat patients with genotype 1 for only 6 months if the level of viraemia is low was not correct according to our results. This recommendation would lead to a reduction of 18% of the sustained response rate obtained by the 48-week regimen.

Suggested algorithm for the treatment (Figure 21.1)

Finally, our recommendation was to treat naïve patients with ribavirin-interferon combination for 24 weeks and to test the HCV PCR at this point.

If HCV RNA is undetectable, the decision to continue the combination for 24 weeks or not should be taken according to the number of favourable factors (see Figure 20.3). It seems reasonable to stop treatment in case of the presence of almost all the favourable factors, ie, four or five factors. For patients with fewer than four factors, who represent 46% of the population, it seems useful to continue the treatment for a total of 48 weeks.

For patients who remain PCR positive at 24 weeks the choice of whether to treat for 24 weeks or 48 weeks has not been fully resolved. From the perspective of HCV eradication, the combination can be stopped at 24 weeks because the probability of obtaining a sustained virological response is 2%. The remaining question concerns the usefulness of continuing treatment to reduce histological damage, since interferon and ribavirin have not only antiviral, but also antifibrotic and immunomodulatory effects.[8,42] Studies are needed to assess whether patients who fail to respond to combination therapy will benefit from either long-term interferon monotherapy or combination therapy. In patients with detectable HCV RNA after 24 weeks of interferon monotherapy a randomized trial showed that maintenance therapy for 48 weeks improves necrosis and inflammation

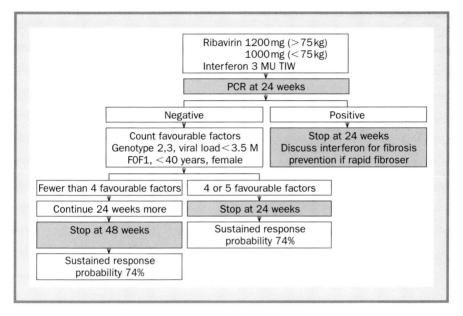

Figure 21.1
Proposed treatment regimen algorithm according to response factors.

in comparison with controls.[44] A proposed algorithm for follow-up is given in Figure 21.2.

Usefulness of genotype and viral load determinations

For patients who remain PCR positive after 24 weeks of ribavirin-interferon, there is no need to determine the genotype or perform any quantitative measurement before or during treatment. The combination can be stopped whatever the response factors. In contrast, for patients who are PCR negative at 24 weeks, clinicians need to know the genotype and the baseline viral load to decide whether to continue treatment for an additional 24 weeks. ALT, PCR, or viral-load measurements at 4 weeks or 12 weeks are not useful. However, for the very high-risk group (men, older than 40 years and with at least septal fibrosis, F2) therapy should be continued whatever their viral characteristics.

From these results it was reasonable to recommend 48 weeks of treatment only for patients who are PCR negative at 24 weeks and who do not have four or five favourable response factors.

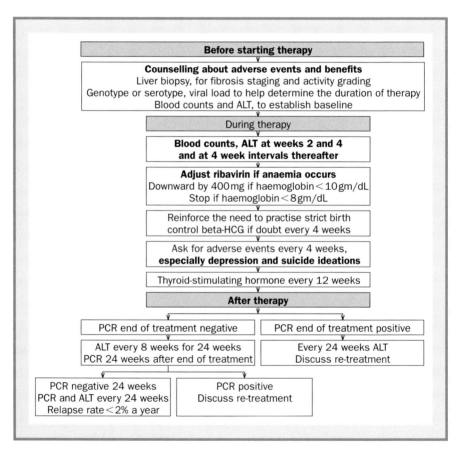

Figure 21.2
Proposed follow-up of treated patients.

Efficacy of pegylated interferon

22

Rational

Pegylation of proteins decreases clearance and thereby increases half life and to some extent biological activity. The pegylated interferons, either alfa-2b or alfa-2a, have shown pharmacokinetic profiles allowing one injection per week (Figure 22.1).[45,46]

Efficacy of pegylated interferon in comparison with standard interferon

Pegylated interferon alfa-2b (0.5, 1.0, and 1.5 µg per kg) has shown a greater efficacy than standard interferon regimen (3 MU TIW) on virological endpoints, particularly at the end of treatment (Figure 22.2).[38] When genotype and viral load were taken into account the efficacy was low in patients with genotype 1 and in patients with high viral load (Figure 22.3).

Pegylated interferon alfa-2a (180 µg or 90 µg once a week) for 48 weeks has shown a greater efficacy than standard interferon regimen (6 MU TIW alfa-2a for 12 weeks and then 3 MU TIW for the remaining 36 weeks of treatment; Figure 22.4).[39,40]

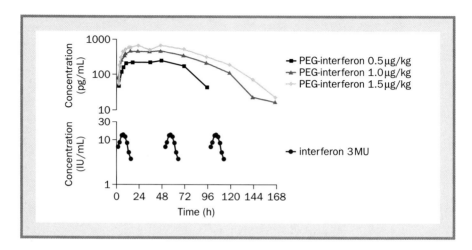

Figure 22.1
Pharmacokinetic single-dose profiles of pegylated interferon alfa-2b versus standard interferon alfa-2b. Adapted with permission.[45]

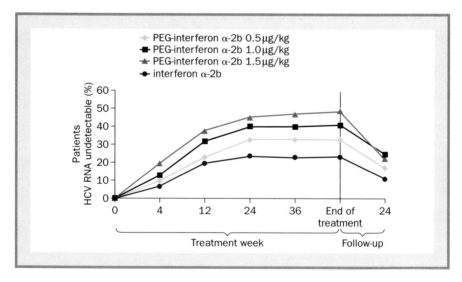

Figure 22.2
Efficacy of pegylated interferon alfa-2b: loss of HCV RNA over time. Adapted with permission.[38]

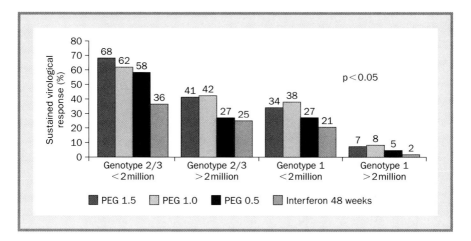

Figure 22.3
Efficacy of pegylated interferon alfa-2b according to genotype and viral load. Adapted with permission.[38]

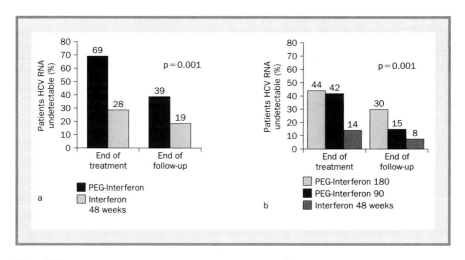

Figure 22.4
Efficacy of pegylated interferon alfa-2a. a) Comparison of PEG 180 with standard interferon. Adapted with permission.[39] *b) Comparison of PEG 180 with PEG 90 and standard interferon in patients with bridging fibrosis or cirrhosis. Adapted with permission.*[40]

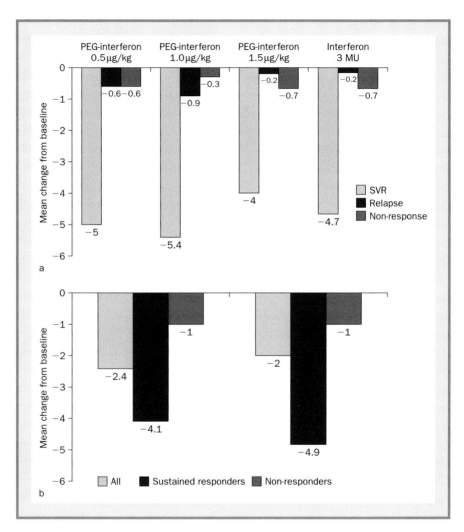

Figure 22.5
Efficacy of pegylated interferons on histological features. a) Pegylated interferon alfa-2b. Inflammation grade expressed by Knodell histological index without fibrosis score. Adapted with permission.[38] b) Pegylated interferon alfa-2a. Knodell histological index included fibrosis score. Adapted with permission.[39]

Efficacy on histological endpoints

There was an improvement in histological endpoints in comparison with baseline values but without difference between PEG interferons and standard interferons (Figure 22.5).[38–40]

Efficacy on extra-hepatic manifestations and on quality of life

There were fewer adverse events in patients receiving lower doses of pegylated interferon alfa-2b in comparison with standard interferon (Figure 22.6).[38]

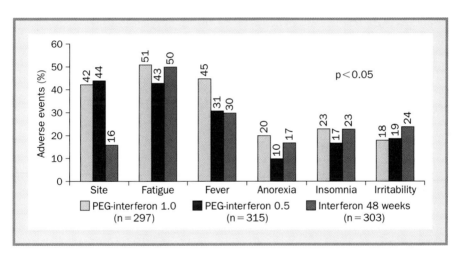

Figure 22.6
Adverse events in patients treated by pegylated interferon alfa-2b. There was significantly less anorexia, insomnia, and irritability in patients receiving PEG 0.5 in comparison with standard interferon. Adapted with permission.[38]

Efficacy of combination with pegylated interferon alfa-2b and ribavirin

23

The optimized combination of interferon alfa-2b 1.5 µg per kg with ribavirin is nowadays the new standard for first-line treatment of naïve patients.

Efficacy on virological endpoints

A randomized trial including 1530 patients has compared three regimens, two combinations of pegylated interferon alfa-2b and ribavirin and the standard ribavirin-interferon combination (Figure 23.1).[41] There was a significant difference in favour of PEG-interferon 1.5 µg per kg combination with ribavirin (Figure 23.2). This arm, contrary to the other groups, had a fixed dose of ribavirin (800 mg) which in retrospective studies was shown to be not the optimum regimen for patients weighing 65 kg or more (Figure 23.3). When the patients receiving the optimized dose (greater than 10.6 mg per kg, that is more than 800 mg a day for a 75 kg person) were compared there was a very significant difference in favour of PEG-interferon 1.5 µg versus standard combination. Among patients infected with genotype-1 HCV there was an increase of sustained response from 33% to 48% (Figure 23.4).

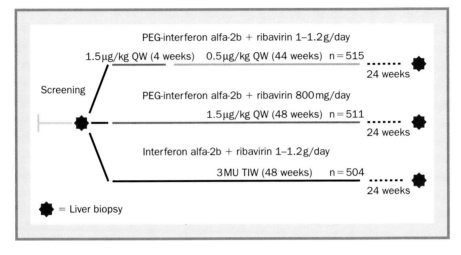

Figure 23.1
Study design of a randomized trial comparing PEG-interferon-ribavirin combination with standard ribavirin-interferon combination. Adapted with permission.[41]

Figure 23.2
Efficacy of PEG-interferon and ribavirin combination. Analysis without adjusting for patient weight. Adapted with permission.[41]

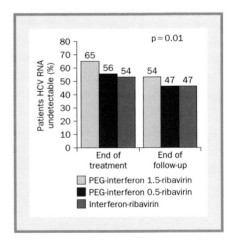

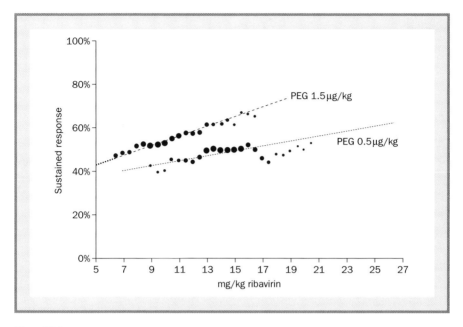

Figure 23.3
Effect of patient weight on sustained virological response when treated by pegylated interferon alfa-2b and ribavirin. Adapted with permission.[41]

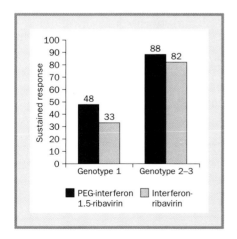

Figure 23.4
Efficacy of PEG-interferon and ribavirin optimized combination. Analysis adjusted on patient weight. Adapted with permission.[41]

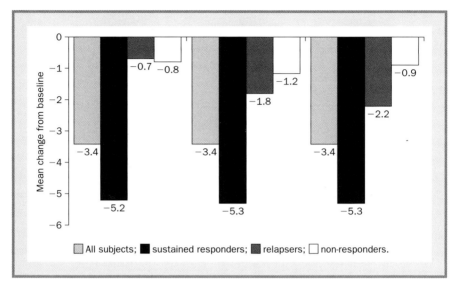

Figure 23.5
Efficacy of combination pegylated interferon alfa-2b and ribavirin on histological features. Adapted with permission.[41] Inflammation grade expressed by Knodell histological index without fibrosis score. A All subjects; B sustained responders; C relapsers; D non-responders.

Factors associated with response

The same factors were associated with non-response and relapse[41] as for standard combination.[37] Therefore post-approval studies must now establish one "à la carte" regimen for optimized combination.

Efficacy on histological endpoints

There were no differences between regimens (Figure 23.5).

Management of relapsers and non-responders

24

Relapsers

A relapser is defined as a patient with undetectable HCV RNA in the serum at the end of the treatment but detectable afterwards. When this treatment was interferon, randomized trials have shown that ribavirin-interferon 24 weeks combination permitted 55% of sustained response versus 5% in patients retreated by interferon alone.[37]

If relapse occurs after ribavirin-interferon combination the best strategy presently is to treat with the optimized combination of PEG-interferon 1.5 µg per kg and ribavirin adjusted on weight. If relapse occurs after the optimized combination ribavirin-interferon the best strategy is unknown: longer duration or tri-therapy with amantadine could be discussed.

Non-responders

A non-responder is defined as a patient with HCV RNA still detectable in the serum at the end of the treatment. A non-responder after interferon alone (24 or 48 weeks) or after the combination ribavirin-standard-interferon should be treated

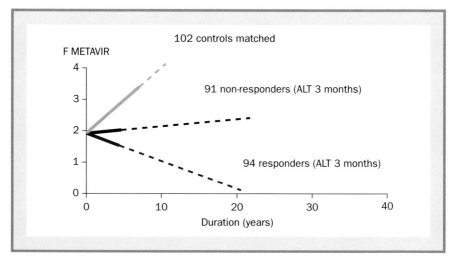

Figure 24.1
Suppressive (or maintenance) concept. Interferon reduces the fibrosis progression among viral non-responders in comparison with spontaneous progression without treatment. Interferon was given for 24–48 weeks in total, without stopping treatment if ALT was still elevated after 3 months of treatment. Adapted with permission.[8]

by the optimized combination of PEG-interferon 1.5 µg per kg and ribavirin adjusted on weight.

In non-responders after the optimized combination ribavirin-interferon for at least 24 weeks the best strategy is unknown. These patients should be included in randomized trials. If it is not possible one option is to treat the patients with extensive fibrosis by PEG-interferon alone to decrease the progression rate to cirrhosis, while waiting for a new generation of drugs. A small dose of PEG-interferon, ie 0.5 µg, is interesting in this case because of its good tolerance and once-a-week injection regimen. This concept of maintenance (suppressive therapy) has been developed with standard interferon monotherapy[8,44,47,49] showing in non-responders a decrease in fibrosis progression rates (Figure 24.1) and an improvement in necrosis and inflammation (Figure 24.2). Maintenance therapy with interferon should probably be repeated, because after cessation of interferon fibrosis progression is restarted (Figure 24.3).

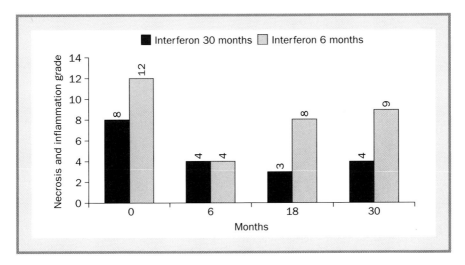

Figure 24.2
Histological benefit of maintenance therapy with interferon. Virological non-responders to 6 months interferon were randomized to 24 more months (maintenance therapy, n = 27) versus no more treatment (n = 26). There was a significant histological improvement in patients receiving maintenance therapy. Adapted with permission.[44]

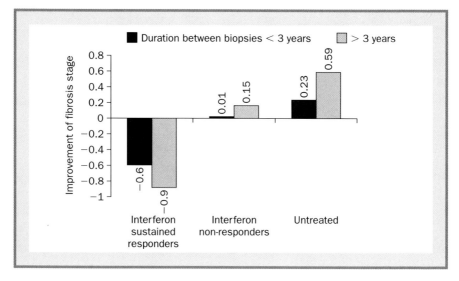

Figure 24.3
Suppressive (or maintenance) concept. Interferon improved the fibrosis stages both in viral responders and in viral non-responders in comparison with untreated patients. When duration between biopsies was longer than 3 years the improvement was greater in sustained responders. In viral non-responders fibrosis progression restarted after 3 years. In untreated patients fibrosis progression was time dependent. Adapted with permission.[47]

Management of patients with cirrhosis

25

Interferon alone

Overviews of randomized trials clearly show that compensated cirrhosis belongs to the full indication of interferon treatment.[33,34] Although lower than in non-cirrhotic patients, there is a significant improvement versus control in randomized trials for ALT response at the end of the treatment (20%), for the sustained ALT response (13%), and for histological response, which can reach 80% for 18 months duration. The effect on HCV RNA seems even better than that observed for ALT. From these results and taking into account the severity of the disease, we think that it is mandatory to treat these patients, because the tolerance is roughly similar to that in non-cirrhotic patients. Interferon is able to reduce by 16% the 4-year mortality rate and by 13% the incidence of hepatocellular carcinoma.[33,34,50,51] The number of randomized studies is small but the meta-analysis of controlled retrospective studies with many more patients are impressive, showing the same reduction in hepatocellular carcinoma and mortality (Figure 25.1; Table 25.1).[51,52]

The results of PEG-interferon in patients with extensive fibrosis or cirrhosis are also very encouraging.[40]

Table 25.1 Risk factors for hepatocellular carcinoma in 2400 patients treated by interferon. Adapted with

Type of response to interferon	Risk ratio	p
Virological		
Sustained	0.20	<0.001
Non-sustained	0.63	<0.001
Biochemical ALT		
Sustained	0.20	<0.001
Mildly elevated	0.36	<0.001
Highly elevated	0.91	Not significant

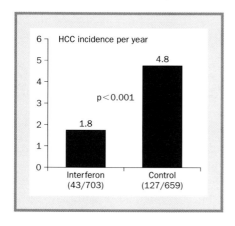

Figure 25.1
Reduction of hepatocellular carcinoma (HCC) incidence following treatment with interferon. Meta-analysis of two randomized controlled trials and five non-randomized controlled trials of interferon in patients with cirrhosis. Adapted with permission.[51]

Combination regimen

In patients with cirrhosis, ribavirin-interferon combination achieved a sustained virological response (below 100 copies per mL 6 months after the end of the treatment) in 20% by the combination versus 5% by interferon alone (P = 0.01) (Figure 25.2).[35,36,53] Optimized

combination of PEG-interferon 1.5 µg per kg and ribavirin in patients with compensated cirrhosis is logically the new first-line treatment with 55% of sustained response rate (24 out of 44; Figure 25.3).[41] Interferon toxicity on platelets and neutrophils must be carefully monitored.

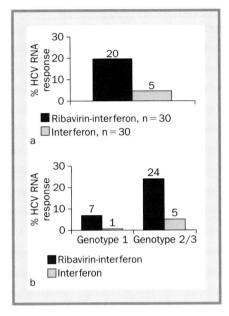

a

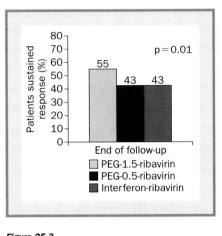

b

Figure 25.3
Efficacy of optimized combination of pegylated interferon and ribavirin in patients with extensive fibrosis or cirrhosis. Adapted with permission.[41]

Figure 25.2
Efficacy of ribavirin-interferon therapy in patients with cirrhosis. Patients were given 1–1.2 g ribavirin plus 3 MU interferon alfa-2 TIW, or 3 MU TIW alone. a) Pivotal randomized trials. b) Pooled European database. Adapted with permission.[35,48]

Management of patients coinfected by HCV and HIV

26

Among patients infected by HIV, HCV coinfection must be systematically screened (anti-HCV antibodies) and treatment of HCV must be discussed when fibrosis is observed at liver biopsy. When transaminase activity is increased in a patient infected by HIV a serum HCV PCR must be administered because false negative of antibodies are possible in immunodepressed patients.

The mean prevalence of HCV antibodies fluctuates between 10% and 30% among a large cohort of patients infected by HIV, 8% among those sexually infected, and 80% among intravenous drug users.

An increase in survival of HIV-infected persons receiving active antiretroviral therapies highlights the problem of chronic hepatitis C. The prevalence of cirrhosis is three-fold higher in HIV-HCV coinfected patients than in HIV-negative HCV-infected patients and one third of coinfected patients are at risk of dying of liver disease.[2,17]

The progression of fibrosis is more rapid in coinfected patients compared to those in matched controls infected by HCV alone. In coinfected patients a low CD4 count ($\leq$200 cells/μL), alcohol consumption ($>$50 g/day), and age at HCV infection are associated with a higher liver fibrosis progression rate.

Anti-HIV treatment is often associated with transaminase increase (D4T, DDI, abacavir, nevirapine, protease inhibitor). When the increase is marked another liver biopsy must be discussed and compared with biopsy before treatment. The following factors can be involved: alcohol consumption, illicit intravenous drug injection, substitution drug toxicity, anti-HIV drug toxicity, coinfection with HBV or Delta virus, liver opportunistic infection, immune restoration, and sclerosing cholangitis. The impact of immune reconstitution on liver fibrosis progression is unknown. However, we have observed a slower fibrosis progression rate in patients receiving anti-protease than in patients not receiving anti-protease. This difference persisted after adjustment for confounding factors.[54]

According to the very severe natural history the most effective treatment of hepatitis C should be given to coinfected patients. Results and tolerance are similar to those of patients infected by HCV only but the benefit-risk ratio is probably higher.[54,55]

Discussion of hepatitis C treatment in a patient coinfected by HIV and HCV

1. If the patient is not treated for HIV and there is no indication for this treatment: a treatment by ribavirin-PEG interferon combination could be given. This strategy is more often discussed in conjunction with a 60% overall sustained response rate.

2. If the patient is not treated for HIV and there is an indication for this treatment: the treatment of HIV must be given without concomitant treatment of HCV. Treatment of HCV can start 6 months later after a good immune and HIV response.

3. If the patient is under treatment for HIV, the treatment of HCV can start when a good immune and HIV response have been obtained.

4. If a patient has a very rapid progression of liver fibrosis with a risk of cirrhosis in the short-term, the treatment of HCV should be discussed in association with anti-HIV treatment, even if the response to HIV treatment is partial.

5. Alcohol consumption should be prohibited in all coinfected HIV-HCV patients because of the rapid fibrosis progression to cirrhosis.

Management of HCV infection after liver transplantation

27

Cirrhosis as a result of HCV is, with alcoholic cirrhosis, the most common indication for orthotopic liver transplantation (OLT) worldwide. After OLT, HCV RNA universally reappears with detectable HCV RNA and 50% to 80% of transplant recipients develop clinical graft hepatitis[56] with probably a more rapid fibrosis progression rate than in non-transplanted patients.[57]

There is a consensus for treating patients with recurrence and fibrosis progression and to reduce immunosuppressive therapy. After recurrence the combination of interferon and ribavirin is effective with an acceptable tolerance[58–60] and hopefully combination with PEG-interferon will increase this efficacy. There is probably an increased risk of haemolysis and anaemia associated with ribavirin in these patients.[59]

There are no clearly defined markers with high predictive values to identify candidates for prophylactic treatment. Interferon monotherapy is effective for prevention of recurrence (Figure 27.1)[61] and trials of PEG-interferon and ribavirine trials are needed according to an encouraging pilot trial of combination (Table 27.1).[62]

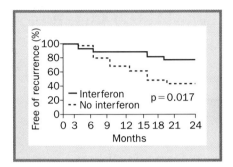

Figure 27.1
Efficacy of interferon alfa-2b in the prophylaxis of recurrent hepatitis C after liver transplantation. Adapted with permission.[61]

Table 27.1 A pilot trial of combination ribavirin and interferon alfa-2b in the prophylaxis of recurrent hepatitis C after liver transplantation. Adapted with permission.[62] 21 patients were included (19 genotype 1b) and were treated within 3 weeks of transplantation and for 48 weeks.

Clinical events	Number of patients
Acute graft hepatitis	4 (19%)
Persistent hepatitis	3 (14%)
Chronic active hepatitis	1 (5%)
Cirrhosis	0 (0%)
No evidence of hepatitis	17 (81%)
HCV RNA-seroconversion	9 (43%)
1-year survival	20 (95%)
Dose reduction	9 (43%)

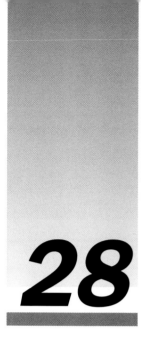

Safety of standard interferon and ribavirin

28

Patients should be fully informed of the potential adverse events before starting therapy.

Severe adverse events

For interferon the main severe adverse events are depression, suicidal ideation, suicide, and sustained hypothyroidia. For ribavirin the main severe adverse events are anaemia and teratogenic effects. There is a 3 g/dL mean drop in haemoglobin concentration occurring in the first 4 weeks of treatment (Figure 28.1). Blood-cell count must be checked at least 2 weeks and 4 weeks after starting therapy and every 4 weeks thereafter. In case of haemoglobin lower than 10 g/dL ribavirin should be reduced by 50%. In case of haemoglobin lower than 8 g/dL ribavirin should be stopped.

Frequent adverse events

For interferon the most frequent adverse events are flu-like symptoms and alopecia. For ribavirin the most frequent adverse events are anaemia, and less frequently pharyngitis, insomnia, dyspnoea, pruritus, rash, nausea, and anorexia (Table 28.1).

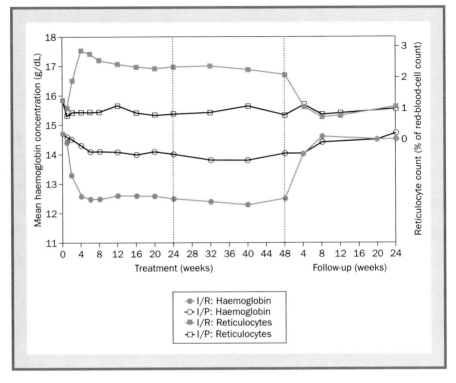

Figure 28.1
Impact of ribavirin-interferon on haemoglobin and reticulocytes count in patients treated by interferon and ribavirin.

Uncommon and rare adverse events

Side-effects occurring in less than 2% of patients treated by combination therapy include autoimmune disease (especially thyroid disease), severe bacterial infections, marked neutropenia, seizures, retinopathy with microhaemorrhages, hearing loss, and tinnitus.

Contraindication to treatment

Contraindications to interferon alfa therapy include psychosis, severe depression, active substance or alcohol abuse, severe heart

Table 28.1 *Adverse events (%) observed in randomized trials.*

	24 weeks		48 weeks	
	Interferon/ ribavirin	Interferon/ placebo	Interferon/ ribavirin	Interferon/ placebo
Discontinuation for adverse events	8	9	21	14
Dose reduction for anaemia	7	0	9	0
Dose reduction for other adverse events	13	12	17	9
Flu-like symptoms				
Fatigue	68	62	70	72
Headache	63	63	67	66
Myalgia	61	57	64	63
Fever	37	35	41	40
Arthralgia	30	27	33	36
Musculoskeletal pain	20	26	28	32
Psychiatric symptoms				
Insomnia	39	27	39	30
Depression	32	25	36	37
Irritability	23	19	32	27
Impaired concentration	11	14	14	14
Anxiety	10	9	18	13
Suicidal ideation	0.6	0.4	2.6	0.2
Attempted suicide	0.2	0	0.2	0
Gastrointestinal symptoms				
Nausea	38	35	46	33
Anorexia	27	16	25	19
Diarrhoea	18	22	22	26
Abdominal pain	15	17	14	20
Dyspepsia	14	6	16	9
Dermatological symptoms				
Alopecia	28	27	32	28
Pruritus	21	9	19	8
Rash	20	9	28	8
Inflammation at injection site	13	10	12	14
Respiratory tract symptoms				
Dyspnoea	19	9	18	10
Cough	15	5	14	9
Pharyngitis	11	9	20	10

disease, severe neutropenia or thrombocytopenia, organ transplantation (except liver), decompensated cirrhosis, uncontrolled seizures, pregnancy, and non-reliable methods of contraception. In fact, with the advice of a psychiatrist it is sometimes possible to treat patients with psychosis or depression. Patients with bone marrow compromise or cytopenias, such as neutrophils below 1000 and below 75 000 platelet count per mL should be treated cautiously with frequent monitoring of cell counts. Relative contraindications are uncontrolled diabetes and uncontrolled autoimmune disorders (such as rheumatoid arthritis, lupus erythematosus, psoriasis and thyroiditis).

Absolute contraindications to ribavirin are pregnancy, unreliable methods of contraception, haemodialysis, end-stage renal failure, severe anaemia, and haemoglobinopathies. Relative contraindications are medical conditions in which anaemia can be dangerous, especially coronary heart disease and cerebrovascular disease. Fatal myocardial infarctions and strokes have been reported during combination therapy. Patients with a pre-existing haemolysis or anaemia (haemoglobin <11 g per dL) should not receive ribavirin (Table 28.2).

Table 28.2 Contraindications to treatment with interferon-ribavirin.

Absolute contraindications to interferon	Relative contraindications to interferon
Psychosis*	Bone marrow compromise cytopenia
Severe depression*	eg neutrophils <1000/mL
Substance or alcohol abuse	platelets <75 000/mL
Severe heart disease	Uncontrolled diabetes
Severe neutropenia or thrombocytopenia	Uncontrolled autoimmune disease, eg
Organ transplantation (except liver)	rheumatoid arthritis
Decompensated cirrhosis	SLE
Uncontrolled seizures	psoriasis
Pregnancy	arthritis
Unreliable methods of contraception	

Absolute contraindications to ribavirin	Relative contraindications to ribavirin
Pregnancy	Medical conditions in which common
Unreliable methods of contraception	anaemia can be dangerous, especially
Haemodialysis	coronary heart disease and cerebrovascular
End-stage renal failure	disease**
Severe anaemia (haemoglobin <11 g/dL)	
Haemoglobinopathies	

* With the advice of a psychiatrist, it is sometimes possible to treat patients with psychosis or severe depression.
** Fatal myocardial infarctions and strokes have been reported during combination therapy.

Safety of pegylated interferon and ribavirin

29

The adverse events profiles of PEG-interferon alfa-2b plus ribavirin and standard interferon plus ribavirin were similar. There were no new or unique adverse events.

There was an increase incidence (greater than 5%) in flu-like symptoms in the PEG-interferon 1.5 μg/kg group compared with standard interferon.[41] As previously reported with PEG-interferon monotherapy there was a significant increase in injection-site reaction. This reaction was generally mild, with a localized erythema, and not treatment limiting.

The impact of ribavirin dose optimization was minor, with few more frequent adverse events (>5% difference) in the optimized group for asthenia, cough, and alopecia. A decrease in haemoglobin to less than 10 g/dL occurred in 14% of the optimized combination. A dose reduction for neutropenia (less than 750×10^9 per L) occurred in 21% of the optimized combination, with less than 1% of discontinuation (less than 500×10^9 per L).

The profiles of neutrophils, platelets and haemoglobin during treatment is described in Figure 29.1.

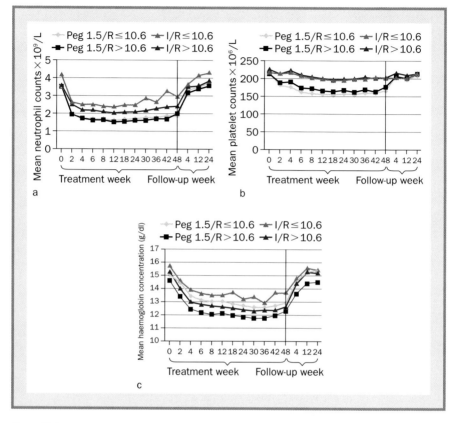

Figure 29.1
Impact of optimized pegylated interferon and ribavirin combination on neutrophils (a), platelets (b), and haemoglobin (c). Adapted with permission.[41]

Who needs to be treated and how to explain the goals to the patient

30

An algorithm for the treatment decision is presented in Figure 30.1. When one considers the natural history of hepatitis C there are three different goals for the treatment: to prevent the occurrence of cirrhosis and its complications; to reduce the extra-hepatic manifestations; and to prevent the contamination of other people (ie, surgeon or drug user).

Is there a group of patients for whom the treatment is useless?

If the patient is not at risk of progressing to cirrhosis, has no symptoms, and is not at risk of transmitting the virus there is no need to treat (ie, 60 years old asymptomatic individual contaminated 30 years ago and without fibrosis at biopsy). Patients without any fibrosis (METAVIR F0) represent only 7% of a study on 4552 patients.

If the patient has decompensated cirrhosis the benefit of treatment is unknown. Because of adverse events, and particularly leucopenia, interferon and ribavirin are not presently recommended. Prospective trials are needed with these patients, especially before transplantation.

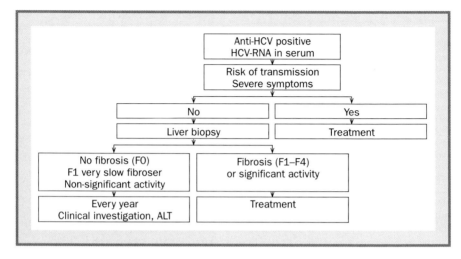

Figure 30.1
Algorithm for treatment decision.

What is the cost-effectiveness of combination regimen?

31

Treatment of hepatitis C is effective and costly. Hepatitis C and its complications are even more costly. Therefore combination regimen is cost effective compared with other widely accepted medical interventions (Tables 31.1–31.5).[63–65]

Table 31.1 Direct medical cost of diagnosis.

Diagnostic test	Cost in Euros (from mean French prices)	Cost in US dollars (from US government mean reimbursement prices (private prices))
ALT	€7	US$9
LISA test	€20	US$27
HCV PCR	€40	US$37
Viral load	€70	US$80 (US$150)
Genotype	€100	Not approved (US$250)
Liver ultrasonography	€60	US$100 (US$240)
Liver biopsy	€500	US$370 (US$1000)

Table 31.2 Direct medical cost of treatment.

Treatment	Drug cost in Euros (from mean French prices)	Drug cost in US dollars (from mean US prices)	Monitoring cost in US dollars (from mean US prices)
48 weeks interferon alone	€3000	US$5000	US$1300
48 weeks ribavirin-interferon	€10 000	US$16 000	US$1100

Table 31.3 Direct medical cost of disease (office visits, lab tests, medications other than interferon or ribavirin, hospitalization). Adapted with permission.[63,64]

Disease	Average cost in Euros for a year (mean French prices)	Average cost in US dollars for a year (mean US prices)
Chronic hepatitis without cirrhosis	€100	US$300
Non-complicated cirrhosis	€1500	US$400
Complicated cirrhosis	€11 000	US$22 000
Hepatocellular carcinoma	€10 000	US$14 000
Transplantation, 1st year	€75 000	US$270 000
Transplantation, successive years		US$26 000

Table 31.4 Cost-effectiveness of combination therapy. Comparison of cost and gain in life expectancy versus coronary artery bypass surgery. Adapted with permission.[65]

	Cost	Gain in life expectancy
Combination regimen	$10 000	3.0 years
Coronary artery bypass surgery	$27 000	1.1 years

Table 31.5 Cost-effectiveness of combination therapy. Comparison of cost per quality-adjusted life years versus accepted medical interventions. Adapted with permission.[64]

	Incremental cost per quality-adjusted life years
Combination regimen	$7500
Screening blood donors for HIV	$14 000
Treatment of hypertension (70 years old)	$5300
Treatment of hypertension (40 years old)	$85 000

Practical guidelines for the management of hepatitis C

32

Liver biopsy

PCR HCV RNA testing makes the diagnosis of hepatitis C infection. However, biopsy is necessary for staging the severity of disease (fibrosis stage) and grading the amount of necrosis and inflammation. Biopsy is also helpful in ruling out other causes of liver disease such as alcoholic features, non-alcoholic steatohepatitis, autoimmune hepatitis, medication-induced, coinfection with HBV, HIV or iron overload.

Liver biopsy is helpful to the physician in deciding both on form of therapy and its duration. Biopsy is usually not helpful when cirrhosis is clinically or biologically obvious. Liver biopsy is usually done by intercostal route. In case of clotting disorders a transjugular route is used.

Complications of liver biopsy

From nine large observations, gathering 98 445 cases of liver biopsy, the incidence of severe adverse events was 3.1 per 1000 (95% CI 2.8–3.5) with a 0.3 per 1000 mortality (95% CI 0.2–0.5).[66] Factors associated with severe adverse events and mortality were cirrhosis, patient's age, and presence of liver cancer.

In the next few decades liver biopsy indications should decrease because of the validation of serum markers.[67]

PCR amplification

Using the latest techniques PCR can detect 100 HCV RNA copies per mL of serum. Testing for HCV RNA is a reliable way of demonstrating HCV infection and is the most specific test of infection. Testing HCV RNA is particularly useful: when transaminases are normal; several causes of liver disease are possible (ie, alcohol consumption); in immunosuppressed patients (ie, after transplantation, in HIV coinfected patients); and in acute hepatitis C before occurrence of antibodies.

Enzyme immunoassay

Anti-HCV is detected by enzyme immunoassay. The third generation test is usually very sensitive and very specific. In case of false positive or false negative doubts, the best test for confirmation of HCV infection is HCV RNA PCR. Immunosuppressed patients infected by HCV may test negative for anti-HCV. Antibody is usually present by 1 month after onset of acute illness. Anti-HCV is still detectable during and after treatment, whatever the response and must not be tested again.

Genotype and serotype

There are six genotypes of hepatitis C and more than 50 subtypes. Knowing genotype or serotype (genotype-specific antibodies) is helpful for the ribavirin-interferon treatment duration choice. Genotypes do not change during the course of infection and must not be tested again. Knowing subtypes (ie, 1a versus 1b) is presently not clinically helpful. There is no relation between the severity of the disease (fibrosis stage) and genotypes.

Quantification of HCV RNA in serum

Methods to measure the level of virus in serum use quantitative PCR and a branched DNA (bDNA) test. In the more recent studies the median of viral load ranged from 2 to 4 million copies per mL (Superquant assay, National Genetics Institute, Los Angeles, CA). Knowledge of viral load is helpful for the ribavirin-interferon treatment duration choice. Patients with high initial viral load have higher relapse rates and benefit more from the 48 weeks regimen than patients with lower viral load. Contrary to HIV infection viral load does not correlate to severity of hepatitis (fibrosis progression).

An effort has been made to define clinically relevant HCV RNA loads in standardized international units (IU), for use in routine clinical and research applications based on standardized quantitative assays validated with appropriate calibrated panels.[68] Two hepatitis C virus RNA quantitative assays were already assessed: the Superquant assay (National Genetics Institute, Los Angeles, CA), for which possibly relevant thresholds were established; and the semi-automated Cobas Amplicor HCV Monitor assay version 2.0 (Cobas v2.0, Roche Molecular Systems, Pleasanton, CA) that measures HCV RNA loads in IU/mL. A value of 2 000 000 copies/mL ($6.3 \log_{10}$ copies/mL) with Superquant was converted to nearly 800 000 IU/mL ($5.9 \log_{10}$ IU/mL) and 3 500 000 copies/mL ($6.5 \log_{10}$ copies/mL) to nearly 1 300 000 IU/mL ($6.1 \log_{10}$ IU/mL). To simplify we recommend a decision threshold at 1 000 000 IU/mL ($6.0 \log_{10}$ IU/mL) to tailor the interferon-alfa/ribavirin treatment duration.

Ten key points for understanding the natural history of HCV

1. Almost all the mortality of the disease is related to complications of cirrhosis.
2. There is almost never a spontaneous clearance of the virus in chronic hepatitis.
3. One third of infected patients will probably never progress to cirrhosis. One third will progress without treatment in

around 30 years and one third will progress in less than 20 years.

4. Despite the risk of fibrosis a patient can be treated for extra-hepatic manifestation or to prevent transmission of the virus.
5. Cryoglobulinaemia is very common (40%) and rarely associated with severe symptoms (1% of vasculitis).
6. The viral load and genotype are not related to the severity of the disease.
7. Alcohol consumption greater than four glasses a day accelerates fibrosis progression.
8. Ageing accelerates fibrosis progression particularly after 50 years of age.
9. HIV coinfection and immunosuppression accelerates fibrosis progression.
10. Normal transaminases do not exclude a progression to cirrhosis even if the risk is less than among patients with elevated transaminases.

Ten key points for understanding HCV treatment

1. There are two goals for the treatment of hepatic manifestation: the first goal is to eradicate the virus; if the virus is not eradicated the second role is to prevent the progression to cirrhosis and the complications of cirrhosis.
2. When a sustained viral response is obtained (negative PCR 6 months after

the end of treatment) the late relapse rate is lower than 5% 4 years later.

3. When a sustained viral response is obtained there is a dramatic improvement of liver histology including necroinflammatory features in all patients and fibrosis stage in non-cirrhotic patients.

4. When a sustained viral response is obtained in cirrhotic patients, a few randomized trials and several retrospective studies observed that the incidence of complications were decreased in comparison to non-treated patients.

5. When a sustained viral response is not obtained, there is a controversy concerning the benefit of treatment. Randomized trials and modelling have shown in these patients an improvement of transaminase activity, viral load, necroinflammatory lesions, and fibrosis progression in comparison with the natural history.

6. The long-term impact of treatment on extra-hepatic manifestations is unknown. Health-related quality of life is improved after treatment in sustained responders.

7. During treatment the quality of life of the patient is generally worse than before because of the adverse events but improves thereafter in sustained responders.

8. Depression and suicide are the most extreme adverse events of interferon.

9. Anaemia and teratogenicity are the most dreadful adverse events of ribavirin.

10. After treatment all adverse events disappeared with the exception of dysthyroidia in less than 3%.

References

1   WHO. Hepatitis C: global prevalence. *Wkly Epidemiol Rec* 1997;
   72: 341–44.

2   Darby SC, Ewart DW, Giangrande PLF, et al. Mortality from
   liver cancer and liver disease in haemophilic men and boys given
   blood products contaminated with hepatitis C. *Lancet* 1997; **350**:
   1425–31.

3   El-Serag HB, Mason A. Rising incidence of hepatocellular
   carcinoma in the United States. *N Engl J Med* 1999; **34**: 745–50.

4   Deuffic S, Buffat L, Poynard T, Valleron AJ. Modeling the
   hepatitis C virus epidemic in France. *Hepatology* 1999; **29**:
   1596–601.

5   Deuffic S, Poynard T, Valleron AJ. Correlation between HCV
   prevalence and hepatocellular carcinoma mortality in Europe. *J
   Viral Hepatitis* 1999; **6**: 411–13.

6   Alter MJ, Kruszon-Moran D, Nainan OV, et al. The prevalence
   of hepatitis C virus infection in the United States, 1988 through
   1994. *N Engl J Med* 1999; **341**: 556–62.

7   Poynard T, Bedossa P, Opolon P, for the OBSVIRC,
   METAVIR, CLINIVIR and DOSVIRC groups. Natural history
   of liver fibrosis progression in patients with chronic hepatitis C.
   Lancet 1997; **349**: 825–32.

8   Sobesky R, Mathurin P, Charlotte F, et al. Modeling the impact
   of interferon alfa treatment on liver fibrosis progression in chronic
   hepatitis C: a dynamic view. *Gastroenterology* 1999; **116**: 378–86.

9 Knodell KG, Ishak KG, Black WC, et al. Formulation and application of a numerical scoring system for assessing histological activity in asymptomatic chronic active hepatitis. *Hepatology* 1981; **1**: 431–35.

10 Ishak K, Baptista A, Bianchi L, et al. Histological grading and staging of chronic hepatitis. *J Hepatol* 1995; **22**: 696–99.

11 The METAVIR cooperative group. Inter- and intra-observer variation in the assessment of liver biopsy of chronic hepatitis C. *Hepatology* 1994; **20**: 15–20.

12 Bedossa P, Poynard T. An algorithm for the grading of activity in chronic hepatitis C: the METAVIR Cooperative Study Group. *Hepatology* 1996; **24**: 289–93.

13 Paradis V, Mathurin P, Laurent A, et al. Histological features predictive of liver fibrosis in chronic hepatitis C infection. *J Clin Pathol* 1996; **49**: 998–1004.

14 Yano M, Kumada H, Kage M, et al. The long term pathological evolution of chronic hepatitis C. *Hepatology* 1996; **23**: 1334–40.

15 Datz C, Cramp M, Haas T, et al. The natural course of hepatitis C virus infection 18 years after an epidemic outbreak of non-A, non-B hepatitis in a plasmapheresis centre. *Gut* 1999; **44**: 563–67.

16 Poynard T, Ratziu V, Charlotte F, et al. Rates and risk factors of liver fibrosis progression in patients with chronic hepatitis C. *J Hepatol* (in press).

17 Wiley TE, McCarthy M, Breidi L, et al. Impact of alcohol on the histological and clinical progression of hepatitis C infection. *Hepatology* 1998; **28**: 805–09.

18 Benhamou Y, Bochet M, Di Martino V, et al. Liver fibrosis progression in human immunodeficiency virus and hepatitis C virus coinfected patients: the Multivirc Group. *Hepatology* 1999; **30**: 1054–58.

19 Bissell DM. Sex and hepatic fibrosis. *Hepatology* 1999; **29**: 988–89.

20 Poynter ME, Daynes RA. Peroxysome proliferator-activated receptor α activation modulates cellular redox status, represses nuclear factor-kB signaling, and reduces inflammatory cytokine production in ageing. *J Biol Chem* 1998; **273**: 32833–41.

21 Pol S, Fontaine H, Carnot F, et al. Predictive factors for development of cirrhosis in parenterally acquired chronic hepatitis C: a comparison between immunocompetent and immunocompromised patients. *J Hepatol* 1998; **29**: 12–19.

22 De Moliner L, Pontisson P, De Salvo GL, et al. Serum and liver HCV RNA levels in patients with chronic hepatitis C: correlation with clinical and histological features. *Gut* 1998; **42**: 856–60.

23 Roffi L, Ricci A, Ogliari CJ, et al. HCV genotypes in Northern Italy: a survey of 1368 histologically proven chronic hepatitis C patients. *J Hepatol* 1998; **29**: 701–06.

24 Mathurin P, Moussalli J, Cadranel JF, et al. Slow progression rate of fibrosis in hepatitis C virus patients with persistently normal alanine transaminase activity. *Hepatology* 1998; **27**: 868–72.

25 Gumber SC, Chopra SC. Hepatitis C: a multifaced disease. Review of extrahepatic manifestations. *Ann Intern Med* 1995; **123**: 615–20.

26 Cacoub P, Poynard T, Ghillani P, et al. Extrahepatic manifestations in patients with chronic hepatitis C. *Arthritis Rheum* 1999; **42**: 2204–12.

27 Zuckerman E, Zuckerman T, Levine AM, et al.

Hepatitis C virus infection in patients with B-cell non-Hodgkin lymphoma. *Ann Intern Med* 1997; **127**: 423–28.

28 Marcellin P, Pouteau M, Benhamou JP. Hepatitis C virus infection, alpha interferon therapy and thyroid dysfunction. *J Hepatol* 1995; **22**: 364–69.

29 Foster GR, Goldin RD, Thomas HC. Chronic hepatitis C virus infection causes a significant reduction in quality of life in the absence of cirrhosis. *Hepatology* 1998; **27**: 209–12.

30 Rodger AJ, Jolley D, Thompson SC, et al. The impact of diagnosis of hepatitis C virus on quality of life. *Hepatology* 1999; **30**: 1299–301.

31 Bonkovsky HL, Woolley JM, and the Consensus Interferon Study Group. Reduction of health-related quality of life in chronic hepatitis C and improvement with interferon therapy. *Hepatology* 1999; **29**: 264–70.

32 Ware JE, Bayliss MS, Mannocchia M, Davis GL. Health-related quality of life in chronic hepatitis C: impact of disease and treatment response: the Interventional Therapy Group. *Hepatology* 1999; **30**: 550–55.

33 Poynard T, Leroy V, Cohard M, et al. Meta-analysis of Interferon randomized trials in the treatment of viral hepatitis C: effects of dose and duration. *Hepatology* 1996; **24**: 778–89.

34 Thevenot T, Regimbeau C, Ratziu V, et al. Meta-analysis of interferon randomized trials in the treatment of viral hepatitis C in naive patients: 1999 update. *J Viral Hepat* 2001; **8**: 48–62.

35 Poynard T, Marcellin P, Lee S, et al. Randomised trial of interferon alpha 2b plus ribavirin for 48 weeks or for 24 weeks versus interferon alpha 2b plus placebo for 48 weeks for treatment of chronic infection with hepatitis C virus. *Lancet* 1998; **352**: 1426–32.

36 McHutchison JG, Gordon SC, Schiff ER, et al. Interferon alfa 2b alone or in combination with ribavirin as initial treatment for chronic hepatitis C. *N Engl J Med* 1998; **339**: 1485–92.

37 Poynard T, McHutchison J, Goodman Z, et al. Is an "à la carte" combination interferon alfa-2b plus ribavirin regimen possible for the first line treatment in patients with chronic hepatitis C? *Hepatology* 2000; **31**: 211–18.

38 Trepo C, Lindsay K, Niederau C, et al. Pegylated interferon alfa-2b monotherapy is superior to interferon alfa-2b for treatment of chronic hepatitis C. *J Hepatol* 2000; **32**(suppl 2): 29 (abstr).

39 Zeuzem S, Feinman SV, Rasenack J, et al. Peginterferon alfa-2a in patients with chronic hepatitis C and cirrhosis. *N Engl J Med* 2000; **343**: 1673–80.

40 Heathcote EJ, Shiffman ML, Cooksley WGE, et al. Peginterferon alfa-2a in patients with chronic hepatitis C and cirrhosis. *N Engl J Med* 2000; **343**: 1673–80.

41 Manns MP, McHutchison JG, Gordon SC, et al. PEG-Interferon alfa-2b in combination with ribavirin compared to interferon alfa-2b plus ribavirin for initial treatment of chronic hepatitis C. *Lancet* 2001; (in press).

42 Poynard T, McHutchison J, Davis GL, et al. Impact of interferon alfa-2b and ribavirin on progression of liver fibrosis in patients with chronic hepatitis C. *Hepatology* 2000; **32**: 1131–37.

43 Anon. Consensus statement: EASL international consensus conference on hepatitis C. *J Hepatol* 1999; **30**: 956–61.

44 Shiffman ML, Hofmann CM, Melissa J, et al. A randomized, controlled trial of maintenance interferon therapy for patients with chronic hepatitis C virus and persistent viremia. *Gastroenterology* 1999; **117**: 1164–72.

45 Glue P, Fang JW, Rouzier-Panis R, et al. Pegylated interferon-alpha2b: pharmacokinetics, pharmacodynamics, safety, and preliminary efficacy data: Hepatitis C Intervention Therapy Group. *Clin Pharmacol Ther* 2000; **68**: 556–67.

46 Algranati NE, Sy S, Modi M. A branched methoxy 40 kDa polyethylene glycol (PEG) moiety optimizes the pharmacokinetics (PK) of peginterferon (alpha)-2a (PEG-IFN) and may explain its enhanced efficacy in chronic hepatitis C (CHC). *Hepatology* 1999; **30**(suppl): 109A (abstr).

47 Davis GL, Esteban-Mur R, Rustgi V, et al. Interferon alfa 2b alone or in combination with ribavirin for the treatment of relapse of chronic hepatitis C. *N Engl J Med* 1998; **339**: 1493–99.

48 Schalm SW, Hansen BE, Chemello L, et al. Ribavirin enhances the efficacy but not the adverse effects of Interferon in chronic hepatitis C: meta-analysis of individual patient data from European centers. *J Hepatol* 1997; **26**: 961–66.

49 Shiratori Y, Imazeki F, Moriyama M, et al. Histologic improvement of fibrosis in patients with hepatitis C who have sustained response to interferon therapy. *Ann Intern Med* 2000; **132**: 517–24.

50 Nishiguchi S, Kuroki T, Nakatani S, et al. Randomized trial of effects of interferon alfa on incidence of hepatocellular carcinoma in chronic active hepatitis C with cirrhosis. *Lancet* 1995; **346**: 1051–55.

51 Poynard T, Moussalli J, Ratziu V, et al. Is antiviral treatment (IFN alpha and/or ribavirin) justified in cirrhosis related to hepatitis C virus? *Acta Gastroenterol Belg* 1998; **61**: 431–37.

52 Yoshida H, Shgiratori Y, Moriyama M, et al. Interferon therapy reduces the risk for hepatocellular carcinoma: national surveillance program of cirrhotic and non cirrhotic patients with chronic hepatitis C in Japan. *Ann Intern Med* 1999; **131**: 174–81.

53 Schalm SW, Weiland O, Hansen BE et al. Interferon-ribavirin for chronic hepatitis C with and without cirrhosis: analysis of individual patient data of six controlled trials. *Gastroenterology* 1999; **117**: 408–13.

54. Benhamou Y, Di Martino V, Bochet M, et al. Beneficial effect of protease inhibitor therapy on liver fibrosis in HIV/HCV co-infected patients. *Hepatology* 2001; **30**(suppl): 362A.

55 Zylberberg H, Benhamou Y, Lagneaux JL, et al. Safety and efficacy of interferon-ribavirin combination therapy in HCV-HIV coinfected subjects: an early report. *Gut* 2000; **47**: 694–97.

56 Gane EJ, Portmann BC, Naoumov NV, et al. Long-term outcome of hepatitis C infection after liver transplantation. *N Engl J Med* 1996; **334**: 815–20.

57 Berenguer M, Ferrell L, Watson J, et al. HCV-related fibrosis progression following liver transplantation: increase in recent years. *J Hepatol* 2000; **32**: 673–84.

58 Bizollon T, Palazzo U, Ducerf C, et al. Pilot study of the combination of interferon alfa and ribavirin as therapy of recurrent hepatitis C after liver transplantation. *Hepatology* 1997; **26**: 500–04.

59 Gane EJ, Lo SK, Riordan SM, et al. A randomized study comparing ribavirin and interferon alfa monotherapy for hepatitis C recurrence after liver transplantation. *Hepatology* 1998; **27**: 1403–07.

60 Samuel D, Bizollon T, Feray C, et al. Combination of interferon alfa 2-B plus ribavirin for recurrent HCV infection after liver transplantation. A randomised controlled study. *Hepatology* 2000; **32**: 295A (abstr).

61 Sheiner PA, Boros P, Klion FM, et al. The

efficacy of prophylactic interferon alfa-2b in preventing recurrent hepatitis C after liver transplantation. *Hepatology* 1998; **28**: 831–38.

62 Mazzaferro V, Regalia E, Pulvirenti A, et al. Prophylaxis against HCV recurrence after liver transplantation: effect of interferon and ribavirin combination. *Transplant Proc* 1997; **29**: 519–21.

63 Joliot E, Vanlemmens C, Kerleau M, et al. Analyse coût-efficacité du traitement de l'hépatite chronique C. *Gastroenterol Clin Biol* 1996; **20**: 958–67.

64 Younossi ZM, Singer ME, McHutchison JG, Shermock KM. Cost effectiveness of interferon 2b combined with ribavirin for the treatment of chronic hepatitis C. *Hepatology* 1999; **30**: 1318–24.

65 Wong JB, Poynard T, Ling MH, et al. Cost-effectiveness of 24 or 48 weeks of interferon alpha-2b alone or with ribavirin as initial treatment of chronic hepatitis C: International Hepatitis Interventional Therapy Group. *Am J Gastroenterol* 2000; **95**: 1524–30.

66 Poynard T, Ratziu V, Bedossa P. Appropriateness of liver biopsy. *Can J Gastroenterol* 2000; **14**: 543–48.

67 Imbert-Bismut F, Ratziu V, Pieroni L, et al. Biochemical markers of liver fibrosis in patients with hepatitis C virus infection: a prospective study. *Lancet* 2001; **357**: 1069–75.

68 Pawlotsky JM, Bouvier-Alias M, Hezode C, et al. Standardization of hepatitis C virus RNA quantification. *Hepatology* 2000; **32**: 654–59.

Index

Page numbers in *italic* denote figure legends where there is no textual reference on the same page.